Just Keep Breathing

Just Keep Breathing

South African Birth Stories

compiled and edited by Sandra Dodson
and Rosamund Haden

Parts of the story 'The Waiting Room' were first published as 'What the Blood Remembers' by Sarah Nuttall in *At Risk: Writing On and Over the Edge of South Africa*, edited by Liz McGregor and Sarah Nuttall (Johannesburg: Jonathan Ball, 2007). They are reproduced here by kind permission of Jonathan Ball Publishers.

First published by Jacana Media (Pty) Ltd in 2008

10 Orange Street
Sunnyside
Auckland Park 2092
South Africa
+2711 628 3200
www.jacana.co.za

ISBN 978-1-77009-576-2

Cover design by banana republic
Set in Stempel Garamond 11/14pt
Printed by CTP Book Printers, Cape Town
Job No. 000670

See a complete list of Jacana titles at www.jacana.co.za

Contents

Introduction

Birth stories can be as compelling as thrillers, and not only to the initiated. Passed down from mother to child, exchanged by friends and relatives, related enthusiastically by sleep-deprived strangers with their newborns in tow, they cement social bonds in a unique way.

Stories of birth have particular resonance in South Africa, representing a narrative of the ordinary in a nation marked and shaped by the extraordinary. Intimate, even confessional at times, they describe one of the most fundamental experiences we have in common, regardless of ethnic or socio-economic background. *Just Keep Breathing* brings together a diverse collection of personal accounts of birth by people born or currently living in South Africa. By turns harrowing, hilarious, shocking, brave and poignant, the contributions include stories by both men and women – including a Rwandan refugee, an HIV-positive mother and a surrogate. A predominantly literary collection, with pieces by established writers of various cultural backgrounds, *Just Keep Breathing* also provides a platform for new South African voices.

The experience of birth encompasses much more than the physical act described in detached detail in birth manuals. Overlaying all the stories in this collection are subtle and suggestive narratives dealing with the emotional or psychological context for the birth of a child. Such layers of meaning give these accounts their rich variety. Reflections on relationships, on love and bonding, on loss of different kinds, are an integral part of many pieces. So, too, are meditations on the significance of names and naming, of identity and cultural tradition. The narratives gathered here draw together and distil all these concerns.

Before introducing the pieces, we would like to say a little about the many *unwritten* stories that inspired, informed and often lightened this project. Over its duration we heard anecdotes ranging from the outlandish to the quirkily humorous: accounts of midwives in Atlantis warning pregnant teenagers, '*In soos 'n piesang, uit soos 'n pynappel, my kind!*';[1] of a man burdened with the name 'Fully Dilated'; of a woman committed to the practice of 'lotus birth', who treated her placenta with sea salt and essential oils and carried it around, still attached to her newborn, for several days. We heard about a 1980s home birth that went awry when neighbours heard screams and alerted the police, who arrived heavily armed to find a woman on the verge of giving birth in a candle-lit living room. We heard about a birth in the back of an Uno, and another that took place on a suburban garden path in the early hours of the morning.

But we also heard more disturbing stories. A domestic worker from the Eastern Cape related how she was left to labour alone and unsupported in an understaffed state hospital, observed intermittently by nurses through a small window in the door of the labour ward. She was attended to only in the final stage of labour, as the baby's head began to crown. Alienating experiences like this are commonplace among women whose birth choices are limited by their geographical or economic circumstances. Yet many such women are reluctant or unable to testify to their emotional trauma in writing. Though their stories are not represented here, we would like to feel that this collection gives them some kind of voice.

○

Makhosazana Xaba's piece, from which the collection takes its title, relates how the author's sense of excitement and uncertainty prior to the birth of her daughter in 1992 coincided with broader apprehensions regarding South Africa's political future:

> The country was poised in uncertainty. So was I . . .
> My maternity leave began in the third week of March.

---

1 'In like a banana, out like a pineapple, my child!'

On 15 March I moved into my new home: Number 401, Palm Grove Court, Berea. The referendum date was out: 18 March. The 'Vote Yes' campaign, conducted by De Klerk's National Party, was visible on our streets, in all our public spaces. It could be heard loudly on many of the radio stations I tuned into. Had I owned a TV set, I know I would have seen it on every channel. I remember trying to keep myself busy by cleaning the flat, buying last-minute necessities, focusing on the baby. I walked the streets reading posters that stared down at me. *Vote* Yes *for change*. Breathe in! The conservatives sounded equally loud. *Vote* No. Breathe out! *Vote* Yes *for change*. Breathe in!

Me, I just kept breathing.

And yet many of the personal accounts published here reveal how far we have come from this period of transition and how much further still from the divisive history of apartheid. Albie Sachs's understated postscript to Vanessa September's account draws a moving analogy between the birth of their child and the birth of a more generous, just and emotionally expressive society. Rosamund Haden describes the very different cultural histories that coalesce in her baby son, whose mixed-race identity would have seemed impossible to his great-grandparents. Ronel Herrendoerfer and Anneke Kamfer-Sloman's piece, about the experience of surrogacy, also reveals a very changed society. The surrogate mother is a coloured woman, while the biological mother is white.

Nonetheless, the social and economic inequalities of the apartheid years are still implicit, visible just off stage, in the contextual detail of many of these accounts. An intimate history of birth can be extraordinarily revealing of the very different ways we have experienced the history of our country. Sindiwe Magona describes how, after undergoing a Caesar, she made the journey back to Gugulethu alone, by bus, carrying her new baby and belongings. Seeing her struggling, white passengers made space for her in the 'whites only' section downstairs.

Phillippa Yaa de Villiers's piece interweaves an account of the home birth of her son with her own birth story, describing how the experience of having a child gives her the sense of kinship she has always yearned for. Adopted by a white family in apartheid South Africa, she was to discover at the age of twenty that she had a Ghanaian father and a white Australian mother.

In the context of the rise of HIV/AIDS in South Africa, birth has assumed new meanings that radically redefine its role within a relationship as well as its broader cultural significance. For HIV-positive women, following the ordeal of having a baby, there is the added psychological burden of waiting to find out if their newborn has contracted the virus. Even those fortunate enough to have had access to drugs which help prevent mother-to-child transmission must endure this sort of anxiety post-birth. Nolubabalo Gloria Ncanywa, from the AIDS support group mothers2mothers, writes a brave account of her discovery that she is HIV-positive while pregnant with her second child. From a very different vantage point, the paediatrician Mark Patrick tells of his experience of the devastating impact of HIV. His story describes movingly how his pregnant wife, also a paediatrician, is exposed to the virus while they are treating a critically ill baby in a rural clinic.

The experience of refugees in South Africa is also reflected in this collection. Living on the edge of society, refugee women are among the most marginalised people in the country, and perhaps the least able to make public the ordeal of birth in a strange place, far from family and friends. Along with recollections of homes, jobs and family members they have lost, many also bring with them memories of a son's or daughter's birth in a country that child will possibly never know. Epiphanie Mukasano writes poignantly of her daughter's birth in Rwanda, and of how, at sixteen, she is now unable to pronounce her Rwandan surname. Her mother laments this loss of her daughter's cultural heritage.

Sarah Nuttall and Marita van der Vyver each describe an altogether different kind of loss. In both pieces the birth of a second child is portrayed in moving counterpoint to the traumatic loss of a first-born. Kholeka Sigenu writes with similar dignity about the underlying grief she felt as she nurtured her newborn son. The baby's twin, a daughter, had died soon after their premature birth.

Birthplace has a profound significance in many of these narratives. Alongside 'diaspora' stories, relating the birth experiences of South Africans now living elsewhere, there are pieces, such as Sandra Dodson's, that evoke a yearning to give birth in South Africa after many years abroad. The theme of birthplace is present in other, more local ways, too. Makhosazana Xaba describes how, as a rural midwife in KwaZulu-Natal, she delivered babies in huts, on river banks, or in the back of an ambulance parked next to a footpath, the woman's home being inaccessible by road. In all her years of practice, she never lost a baby or its mother. Ruth Ehrhardt writes how her mother, with no previous experience of midwifery, was called to a remote farm worker's cottage outside Ceres to tend a woman in labour. The woman was afraid to give birth at the local hospital as she had an outstanding bill.

In stark contrast to these accounts, most stories in the collection describe hospital births. Some writers express ambivalence about a medicalised birth environment, while others convey how access to sophisticated medical technology has saved their babies' lives. Colleen Higgs writes about the premature Caesarean delivery of her baby daughter after she developed pre-eclampsia, while Maire Fisher describes her sons, also born by Caesarean section, as 'miracles of medical expertise'. Rahla Xenopoulos, who gives birth to triplets by Caesarean, tells of her sense of detachment as doctors work deftly to remove the intertwined babies. Disputing that there is any such thing as 'natural' birth, Reviva Schermbrucker describes how both her sons would have died if she hadn't had Caesars. Neither of her children, she says, is any the worse for having come out through the 'trapdoor'.

However, in several accounts there are disturbing hints or attributions of medical negligence. Also, stories of home births attended by midwives suggest that for some women a familiar environment is perceived to be far safer than a hospital, where unwanted or unnecessary medical intervention is more likely.

Birth inevitably raises gender issues, as men suddenly find themselves in a marginal, supporting role, and several stories in this collection describe conflict with a partner or husband during pregnancy or labour. Joanne Hichens's piece, written as an ironic take on a soap-opera script, gives hilarious insight into the way birth doesn't always go according to plan. Not going according to plan means, among other things, that in the throes of labour one does not necessarily feel the closeness to one's partner described rosily in the birth manuals. Gender issues of a different kind surface in several other stories. Finuala Dowling draws attention to the predominance of men in the field of obstetrics, and with wry humour questions her 'need' of a male obstetrician. Elleke Boehmer relates amusingly how, in the historically male-dominated academic environment of Oxford, a student struggles to reconcile her tutor's status as mother with that of her status as an academic. And as a lesbian couple wanting children, Susan Newham and Roxi Blake describe their remarkable and sometimes surreal search for a suitable sperm donor.

Until fairly recently, men were prevented from witnessing the birth of their children. Nowadays, it is much more common for them to be present. It therefore seemed important to give men themselves a voice. Sivuyile Mazantsi's piece begins in a tone of jocular detachment, but one senses his growing sympathy and discomfort as his girlfriend is marched down the hospital corridor like 'a prisoner' and tied to the bedframe with her legs splayed. The humorous tone of Troy Blacklaws's and Imraan Coovadia's stories also changes noticeably as the birth of a child evokes unexpectedly powerful feelings.

If men are marginalised on one level, on another they have a central role in the birth experience, being able to observe with an objectivity impossible for women. This accounts for the sometimes shocking visual clarity of Andrew Weeks's piece. Women, on the other hand, often report not being able to remember their experience with accuracy or, alternatively, not being able to find words adequate to it. This 'blind spot' is closely explored by the child psychologist Tanya Wilson, who articulates how the collapse of a symbolic language to make sense of birth in turn threatened her sense of identity as a mother. Similarly, Willemien de Villiers describes how her personal birth story seems 'stuck on some distant battlefield where abandoned fragments of memory lie buried in shallow trenches'. Interweaving a richly symbolic dream narrative about pregnancy and birth with autobiographical passages set in the present, this is the piece closest to pure fiction.

○

Having compiled and edited this collection, we find it surprising that birth is typically regarded as being beyond the pale of the literary. 'Serious' literature almost invariably sidesteps the subject. Its portrayal, outside the scientific language of modern obstetrics, is restricted largely to the popular media, where it is often sensationalised or given sentimental treatment. One of the primary aims of this project is to give literary value to this commonplace but deeply significant experience. The stories collected here show how original and diverse, how funny and profound, representations of birth can be. While opening up new literary territory, they also demystify many of the cultural illusions and residual taboos that surround the subject. Rising to the challenge of 'saying the unsayable', these extraordinarily candid stories now speak for themselves.

Sandra Dodson and Rosamund Haden, Cape Town, March 2008

Midwives, Mothers, Memories

Makhosazana Xaba

In my early twenties, I delivered hundreds of babies. Naturally, my interest in my own birth and that of my daughter tends towards the technical.

Among other things, I wish I knew how long it took me to journey through Mama's birth canal. Was I like most babies, who understand the advantage of approaching the new world head first? Or did I exit feet first? If I came head first, had I turned around a week or two or just before my birth date? What was my Apgar score? I would like to see the record of all this: *5 p.m.: vaginal examination – 8 cm dilated; 5:30 p.m.: membranes rupture; 6 p.m.: pushing begins.* Every single detail!

Theoretically, there is a record of my birth somewhere, because I was one of the fortunate few in the late fifties to have been delivered by a trained midwife: Mama's aunt, Mrs. Sanah Mamashela, fondly called 'Staff' by the community. Oral history has it that she was the first black staff nurse and midwife to ride a bicycle around Mgungundlovana (Greytown). A bicycle-riding, black midwife – Mgungundlovana's own pioneer! The women she helped deliver must have revered her.

Getting hold of those records of my birth would be a treat. I am curious about the kind of records Sanah would have kept in the fifties. How did she monitor labour? What charts did she use? The mere thought of looking at the papers – yellowing, time-crumpled – excites me. Most of all, I wish to see Staff's signature attesting to her professional presence at my arrival.

Sanah passed away in 1999. Now that I think of it, I doubt she would have kept Mama's birth records for so long. In fact, I doubt that she would have made any notes on Mama's labour at all, because technically she was off duty when I arrived. What else can I rely upon? Decades ago, Mama used to tell me the story of my birth, but as her memory, too, has faded (she calls

1

her brain a sieve), she cannot confirm the details I have kept alive in my head. I shall have to trust my recollection, while allowing my imagination to fill some gaps.

But first, Mama and sex. I have always wanted to ask Mama whether she and my father had pleasurable sex when they made me. But I dare not. I am very curious about the answer, though, because I think that some of my demons may originate in the nature of that sex they had sometime in September of the previous year. I believe there is always something we can trace to the nature of the sex our parents had when they conceived us. There has to be.

During Mama's pregnancy my parents, both schoolteachers, were living with my three-year-old brother in kwaMpande, on the outskirts of Pietermaritzburg. As the winter school holiday approached, they discussed visiting Mama's aunt Sanah, whom they had not seen in a long time. Of all their relatives, Sanah lived nearest to them. And so, close to my due date, off they went to Mgungundlovana. Mama helped around the house whenever Sanah was out on her legendary bicycle. Sanah was a mother to five children, and Mama became the parent figure when Sanah was on midwife duty and the men were out. I suspect that my father was often in town, charming willing listeners with his musical deftness and exuberant handling of the three languages he spoke. A raconteur of note, with music running through his veins, he attracted listeners like light attracts moths. Perhaps he also connected with the teachers in the area and in this way found decent drinking places, as teachers would have demanded for themselves. Sanah's husband was also known to love the bottle. The two of them probably painted Mgungundlovana all the colours of the liquids they could find.

When the holiday neared its end, Sanah said to Mama, 'Nomvula, your time is close. You should not go back to kwaMpande. Stay with us until the baby is born.' My parents took Sanah's advice. My father went back home alone.

I imagine that the journey I began on the afternoon of 10 July 1957 was bumpy at times, but on the whole exciting, urgent and desired. I see Staff arriving home wearily, alighting from her bicycle, walking into her home and packing away her midwifery suitcase. Then, just as she is sitting down to a welcome-home cup of tea, Mama – or is it me? – disrupts her routine. And so, on that evening, she becomes midwife Staff in her own home. I imagine the coal stove emitting sparks of heat and warming the whole house, reaching me, too, in the bedroom Mama is using.

Mama said she had short labours. She did not remember, though, exactly when I was born. It was sometime in the evening, on a Wednesday. I was luckier than most, because I was delivered at home. I must have smiled before I was a day old from the sheer exhilaration of a family welcome. What more could a newborn wish for?

Sanah helped Mama as efficiently as she could. A skilled and experienced midwife, she may also have been a little blasé. My birth, though no doubt special to her in some small way, was still a technical delivery. May the bones of her fingers rest in peace! She was there to ensure that Mama's anxiety was reduced to the minimum and that my confidence to complete my crossing was increased to the maximum. My father was absent.

○

While a student midwife, I seldom thought of my grand-aunt Sanah. I wish I could say that she was my role model, that I became a midwife because of her. Dignified as that would have been, my decision was, sadly, a result of indecent laws that limited career choices for black women of my time.

The circumstances of my midwifery experience were different from Sanah's. In the fifties, Sanah was alone, on her bicycle. In the eighties, I was a live-in midwife at a small rural hospital in KwaZulu-Natal, with an ambulance and a driver. I was a member of a small team of midwives.

Over and above the hospital deliveries, we frequently delivered babies in the ambulance, often near some path between the woman's home and the nearest store, kraal, school or church. We delivered others on river banks, in darkly lit huts, near shops often named So-and-so's General Dealer.

The most memorable deliveries were those when the driver and I would arrive at the foot of a hill, park the ambulance and watch a group of men come down the hill with unbelievable dexterity, holding a home-made stretcher of bamboo, grass and wood. The pregnant woman would be lying as comfortably as such a carriage would allow, with blankets over her body. The men would meet us. I would open the ambulance door and greet the woman. The men would put the stretcher inside and leave us alone. Once I had made an assessment and a decision, we either drove back to the hospital or, some time later, I opened the door of the ambulance to waiting family members, stretcher-bearers and passers-by with a new arrival in my hands.

The message that a woman was in urgent need of a midwife would often be given by a boy who had been instructed to run down the hill to make a call to Ekhombe Hospital from the closest general dealer. The system worked. Our ambulance driver knew every single general dealer, school, clinic and church by their names. He knew all the hills and hillocks by their shapes, the rivers by the bends of their banks and the waves of their waters. He knew the roads and paths by the colour of their soil, the forests by the sway of their trees. He knew the kraals by the smell of their dung and the numbers and types of their animals. He knew the valleys by the slants of their slopes and the shadows of their shrubs.

As we drove together, I was captivated time and again by how he could take one look at the clouds and predict when the first raindrops would fall. Or how he could spot newly built anthills and tell the age of old ones. He could establish where we were by looking at the rocks along the road, because he recognised them by their size and the distance between them. He did not need road signs. The few that existed were often faint and hard to read. He knew alternative routes to take on occasions when rivers had burst their banks and made some roads impassable. Not once did we get lost in the vastness of the rural north. Not once did I lose a baby or its mother.

◌

Sixteen years ago I gave birth to my daughter, Nala. When the day came, I felt as confident as I imagine Sanah did. Unlike Mama on the day I arrived, this was my first birth. I also knew it would be my last.

The desire to have a child in my thirties, back home in a country on the brink of political change, had prompted me to visit a gynaecologist, who delivered the news which confirmed my niggling suspicion that I was unable to become pregnant: my Fallopian tubes were blocked.

Methodical to a fault, I moved into action. The journey from a second opinion to further diagnostic tests and then to the operating theatre was swift. Giving his opinion after the surgery, my doctor at Coronation Hospital warned: 'Just remember that you have a maximum of two years to play with. And only one tube.' *Play with* struck a discordant note for me. 'If you are prone to adhesions,' he continued, 'the Fallopian tubes often close again, even after the operation.'

In December 1991, I returned to Johannesburg from KwaZulu-Natal – pregnant, with one suitcase and no place to live. But I wasn't worried. I had taken up a new job at Wits Medical School and moved from one house to the next, house-sitting for holidaymakers. My pregnancy had, until then, been smooth: free of morning sickness and strange cravings. However, I continued to gain so little weight that my Johannesburg General Hospital midwives would ask at each visit, 'Is something worrying you?' I walked the streets of Hillbrow, Berea, Yeoville, inner-city Johannesburg and Parktown, where my office was located. All indications were that it might be some weeks before I would find a place to live. But that didn't bother me. My estimated date of delivery (EDD) was 31 March. I had ample time.

What really did begin to bother me, though, was the whites-only referendum planned for March. No, I wasn't just bothered; the referendum induced a thunderstorm that raged in my head. I instructed the thunder to confine itself to my head, as my abdominal area was out of bounds. It seemed to listen.

The country was poised in uncertainty. So was I. I began to hear stories of people panic buying, stocking foodstuffs and basic necessities. I also heard that some whites were leaving the country. It was around then that I first heard of the popularity of Australia as a destination for white emigrants. The national scales could tip in any direction. So could mine. At work, a colleague suggested that I should insist on being admitted to hospital a day before the referendum. That way, if the majority vote was undesirable, I could plan my departure back into exile within the safety of the hospital walls. Her advice made sense. But having decided against having a child in exile, I was not prepared to leave the country again.

After house-sitting in five homes in five different areas of the city, I found a flat. My maternity leave began in the third week of March. On 15 March I moved into my new home: Number 401, Palm Grove Court, Berea. The referendum date was out: 18 March. The 'Vote Yes' campaign, conducted by De Klerk's National Party, was visible on our streets, in all our public spaces. It could be heard loudly on many of the radio stations I tuned into. Had I owned a TV set, I know I would have seen it on every channel. I remember trying to keep myself busy by cleaning the flat, buying last-minute necessities, focusing on the baby. I walked the streets reading posters that stared down at me. *Vote* Yes *for change*. Breathe in! The conservatives sounded equally loud. *Vote* No. Breathe out! *Vote* Yes *for change*. Breathe in!

Me, I just kept breathing.

On the morning of 30 March, I had three things on my to-do list: watch a movie, collect beanbag cushions from the store and pack a bag to take to hospital. It was the day that I was to take everything slowly, preparing for the next day, my EDD. At the Hillbrow movie theatre, I chose to watch *Boyz N the Hood*. When I left, my mood had changed. I had not been prepared for the film's violence and degradation. And, oh, so much blood! The movie made me sad.

Slowly I walked to the store and arranged for the delivery of my three beanbags, then made my way home. It was five thirty when the delivery van arrived, just as the store manager had said. The items of furniture in my singles flat had increased to five: three beanbags for visitors, a bed for me and my baby, and a bookshelf.

I was bending over one of the beanbags, wiping it down with a wet cloth, when a pain, sudden and extremely sharp, shot through my abdomen. I dropped onto the beanbag, cloth in hand, and automatically looked at my wristwatch. It was forty-five minutes after five, on the dot. Though I had never had labour pains before, I had witnessed enough births to know that this was a powerful contraction. But labour pains are meant to start in a dull and distant sort of way, I thought. Why was this solitary one so severe?

Mama had told me that all her labours were short. Maybe I was to be like Mama. Maybe I was going to have a precipitate labour. No, I couldn't deal with that. But if I had to, I was glad to have the beanbags; I was going to make sure my baby landed softly on one of them. At that thought I rose and quickly finished wiping the first beanbag, then moved on to the second one.

Another contraction, equally strong, struck at six p.m. When that one had passed, I moved on to the third beanbag, and then to the wardrobe to start packing my bag. The next contraction, which hit me while I stood over my travel bag, felt much stronger than the first two. It came after fifteen minutes. Could my labour be a day early?

It began to look as if I was not to spend the night in my flat. I decided to walk upstairs to the domestic workers' quarters to find MaButhelezi, who cleaned the offices at the medical school. She and I were friends, and I needed her to know that I was going into labour. With the authority of a mature woman, she told me that I had the whole night ahead of me.

I had the telephone numbers of four colleagues who had offered to drive me to hospital when my labour began. By the time I had walked down the stairs back to my flat, I did not need to check my wristwatch. I knew the fifteen-minute interval had shortened. I knew I had to hurry to finish everything I needed to do.

I called Mama first, just to let her know. She promised to call again before she went to bed, to check how far I had progressed.

I called the first friend and colleague. The background noise suggested that she was at a party. It's a Monday, I thought. Who parties on Mondays? 'Oh relax,' she laughed. 'You midwives like to panic. I'm sure nothing will happen tonight.' I hung up. By now I was breathing methodically with each contraction. They were as regular as the midwifery books said they would be. *Breathe.*

I called the next colleague, Stephanie Moore. *Breathe.* I gave a brief account of what had happened and said, 'Steph, please come as soon as you can.' *Breathe.* I truly love this baby. *Breathe.* When Stephanie buzzed, it was eight thirty. *Breathe.*

We were at the Johannesburg Hospital's reception area fifteen minutes later. I asked for a wheelchair. Some nurses laughed at me. Another contraction came. I bent over, in agony. A wheelchair appeared. By the time I sat down, the contraction was over and I smiled at the nurses.

'*Ah, wena,* you are still smiling! *Uzawuthi shu ubaselwe-ke*[1] this time,' one of them said.

'Relax, my sister, the night is long,' I heard another one say. I smiled again, but my face metamorphosed as the next contraction came. I noticed a bewildered look on Stephanie's face. I wanted to reassure her that I was fine. But instead I had to ... *breathe.*

'Hey, hey, hey, take this one away, *uzozalel 'ereception*! *Uhamba nawe lomfazi womlungu Sisi?*'[2]

'Yes,' I replied.

'OK, let her finish all the admin. She will come find you that side. *Mhambiseni! Mhambiseni!*'[3]

I kept reminding myself to breathe. I began to doubt that I would last the night. I was taken to the admissions cubicles. A midwife from the cubicle next to mine greeted me. I tried to find a comfortable position, but before I could, my waters broke. I shouted to announce this. A white midwife was in my

---

1 'You have a good reason to suffer ...'
2 'You are going to give birth at Reception. Is this white woman with you?'
3 'Take her away! Take her away!'

cubicle within a split second. With matching speed, her fingers were in my vagina.

'Take her to the labour ward. She is nine centimetres dilated,' she shouted. I saw Stephanie walk through the curtains, my files in her hands. She handed them over to the midwife.

I was surprised. Nine!

'Would you like me to come with you?' Stephanie asked.

'Sure, if you have the time.'

We had both assumed without any discussion that she would bring my files and go back home. We had not thought I would progress so quickly.

As they transferred me by stretcher to the labour room, Stephanie walked swiftly next to me, my travel bag in her hand.

My eyes found a clock on the wall as I was moved from the stretcher to the delivery bed. Twenty minutes after nine. Another midwife, a white woman, entered the room, introduced herself and confirmed that Stephanie had my permission to be there. She then busied herself with the delivery tray. My body busied itself with breathing through each contraction. My mind busied itself differently.

What surprised me was how I seemed to have split in two. I was a midwife as well as a woman in labour. My language changed. I told the midwife to come close because the foetal descent had begun and I was about to push. I moved the blanket off my body. It was half past nine. I pushed. Stephanie held on to the sheets next to my head.

I saw the vaginal opening widen. I saw the head push through with familiar determination. The perineum stretched and thinned, stretched and thinned. I realised that it was too late for a neat episiotomy cut. The head came through, the midwife's hands on it. The tear on the perineum was small. It bled.

The push that got the head out was the hardest and the longest. As the rest of the baby's seemingly large body slipped through, my eyes lifted to find the wall clock. Nine fifty. My baby girl's cry was neither lame nor dramatic. It was simple: healthy.

I turned to find Stephanie's eyes. The midwife put the baby on me, so that her cheek rested on my left breast. While the midwife's hand held on to her, mine rushed to the small of her back. I closed my eyes. I moved the fingers of my right hand, slowly and carefully, up and down her lower spine. I sighed. She was intact. No palpable signs of spina bifida, my greatest fear. My eyes opened to her suckling. She was under five minutes old and trying to suckle! I just smiled . . . and smiled. Then I cried because I did not know how to thank her for being so efficient. I cried because sometimes tears are more eloquent than words. I looked into her face, my hands around her. I just kept looking into her face.

She and I, nothing else mattered.

Like my own father, Nala's was absent when she was born. Unlike mine, hers was not just some kilometres away. He was across the Atlantic Ocean. Unlike her Wednesday-born parents, Nala is a Monday baby.

When Mama called again, it was a quarter to midnight. 'I called your flat first, then the hospital. When they told me that you had already delivered, I did not believe them!' Her smile reached me through the phone line. Mother to mother, we spoke with excitement. She told me that she would book a seat on the Greyhound bus the next day. When we said our goodbyes, it was after midnight. The last day of March 1992 had begun.

The Rhythm of the Beat

Finuala Dowling

Twice I have walked into a room where, only an hour or two before, a baby has been born. In each case, the midwife has just left and the house is still, as if the walls themselves, the very vegetables in their racks, the upturned cups drying beside the sink, have entered into contemplation with the nursing mother, the awed father.

My own experience of birth was nothing like this. I lay on my back beneath a fluorescent light with a foetal monitor strapped around me, etherised from the waist down, pumped full of labour-inducing drugs. I'd been in hospital since nine in the morning, when two student nurses had shaved me and administered an enema. (Birth is disgusting, but they try to do it cleanly.) Now the clock on the delivery room wall said ten to six. Still the baby had not come.

And why should she? In her opinion, she had another five days to go.

I knew precisely the moment of her conception, when her short stint as a zygote ended, when she left the Fallopian tube behind and embedded herself. I know because she announced the moment herself.

In the narrow bed I had just left, my husband's breathing rose and fell steadily, contentedly. I lay awake, adjusting to the cool, unrumpled sheets of the single bed against the opposite wall. It was the December holidays, and we were back in Cape Town in my old family home, in my old room.

For two months I had used no contraception. That night I lay in the dark wondering, when will it happen, this frightening thing that I want so much? That was when she announced herself, made her first riposte in what has now become a lifelong conversation. It was just like her – the crippling, cramping, three-dimensional pain that immobilised me in that moment of implantation and allowed me to see briefly inside my own womb where my darling blastocyst was clamping herself to my uterine wall. My daughter has a big, dramatic personality, vivid and unequivocal, and she entered the world in that same spirit, with a force that I now recognise as uniquely hers. What the Lord said to Jeremiah must be true for all babies: 'Before I formed thee in the belly, I knew thee; and before thou camest forth out of the womb I sanctified thee . . .'

My gynaecologist gave no credit to my story – indeed, though I've tried to read up on the subject, I have found no reference to this phenomenon of pain on conception – and made his own calculations. By his sums, the birth was ten days overdue. He was going away for the weekend, so it made sense to induce the baby on Friday afternoon. (Birth is inconvenient, but they try to do things smoothly.)

It was fear and ignorance that had led me to hand myself over to a gynaecologist in the first place. In the delivery rooms of my imagination, mothers haemorrhaged beside the blue faces of cord-strangled babies. I needed this man, with his ultrasound machine and blood-pressure monitor and stirrups. I needed to place my urine sample on his immaculate reception desk and to sit quietly in his waiting room watching the ankles of my bovine fellows swell. I needed to step fatly onto his scale and watch the red numbers clock up ever higher. I needed him to talk to me as though I had no education or intellect.

I brought all my feelings of inadequacy to bear. How could someone like me make a perfectly formed baby – one with digits, not flippers? How could I, who could hardly make a cake rise, make a life?

I did not ask the doctor these questions. Only my daughter heard them, and for each question she had an answer. At the first ultrasound, her heartbeat pulsed brightly on the screen, so brightly that even the gynaecologist was moved to say, 'A very strong pregnancy.' My proud showgirl flashed at us in her embryonic Morse code: 'No doubt, no doubt, no doubt.' That was her rhythmic beat. 'Beats' – that's what we call her, short for Beatrice.

Despite her reassurance, the moment I stepped out of that office, the doubts returned. Perhaps it was because I was alone during much of my pregnancy – my husband was on sabbatical, first in Canada, then in New Zealand. Living in Pretoria, I was far away from my family. My friends at work had already started their families, and their spare hours were caught up in fetching children from ballet classes and sports matches. I had too much time to conjure up lurid images of birth defects. Or perhaps this is what all pregnant women do: dream that their babies are monsters, the plates of their skulls folded over one another, the facial features fused.

When I thought I could not bear these imaginings any longer, it would be time for another check-up. Then the gynaecologist would show me my baby's extra-large amniotic sac, her straight, railroad-track spine, her perfect four-chamber heart. 'Beat, beat, beat,' she said. 'Don't worry, I know how to do this. I will never pass a science exam in my life, but I will, with absolute infallibility, execute the stages of my own ontology: primitive streak, Hensen's node, primitive groove, trophoblast, primitive palate, limb bud . . .'

She was brave and clever: I was the coward. I even ate the yellow food of cowardice: lemon creams, granadilla-flavoured drinking yogurt, bananas, caramel-coated ice creams. Meanwhile, she quietly built up her longing for red food: meat, tomatoes, strawberries, KitKats (well, the wrappers are red), maybe even pomegranates.

The first time she moved inside me was at a cabaret venue in Greenwich Village. A jazz musician started up on the double bass and Beats quickened at the plangent notes, saying, 'I am here. I like this very much.'

I'd flown to New York to meet up with my husband, whose sabbatical had come to an end. We stayed in a gay hotel because my husband thought that would be fun and cheap, even cheaper than the Chelsea Hotel round the corner. It being a gay hotel, you could have your chest waxed in your room. I may have been the only pregnant woman ever to grace its chi-chi breakfast room. Having married a man who seldom rises before noon, I had my muffin and coffee alone each morning, horribly conspicuous in my heterosexuality.

Not so lonely, though: increasingly, the little person inside kept me company. People had started to see that I wasn't some poor friendless woman dawdling about on her own. We were a couple, awarded that transnational respect that is a pregnant woman's due. I felt that I could go anywhere, do anything. Good Friday Mass in St. Patrick's Cathedral, the Easter Parade, Broadway shows, lemon meringue pie in midnight diners – my daughter still likes that kind of thing. No wonder that for years after her birth, I could not sleep unless I tucked a pillow up close against my middle, mimicking the memory of that companionship.

When I came home, I saw her face – her sweet tip-tilted nose, her enormous eyes – perfectly outlined on the ultrasound screen. Clearly a girl, or an excessively pretty boy. We were in the home stretch now, and my doubts had abated. She gave me two more strong showings (warnings?) of her personality. During the tumultuous applause – a standing ovation, in fact – for an Afrikaans farce in a packed auditorium, she whirled around and around in her amniotic sac. I felt almost afraid for her excitement, my little thespian.

The next occasion was uncanny. My husband had briefly reappeared and we were visiting friends in Johannesburg. Lunch had turned into supper, and day into night, but he would not agree to leave. They were having a marvellous time. The hostess took pity on me and offered me a bed. I woke up after one in the morning, hungry, morose and utterly unamused at the unabated, drunken chatter of my husband and his friends. I lowered myself heavily into an armchair beside them, my legs wide apart for comfort beneath my voluminous and unflattering Indian cotton frock. I'd recently had a haircut that was the full mistake: all my curls shorn off and a dark, shapeless bush left in their place. Unlovely and, as I felt, unloved, I sat there peeling a naartjie and waiting for the next opportunity to announce our departure.

Then one of my husband's friends came and knelt at my feet, speaking urgently and with a strange intimacy: 'You know,

Nuala, most pregnant women look really beautiful: they glow. But you don't.' I didn't react right away. Physical violence and even verbal abuse have played almost no role in my life. They are not part of my make-up. My mother taught me that 'the soft answer turneth away wrath'. I accepted this person's right to insult me – I'd looked in the mirror, after all. But he wasn't satisfied that I understood his meaning, so he added, 'You look really dowdy.'

I know that my arm rose up then, and that my hand, sticky with naartjie juice, firmed and positioned itself so that it had enough leverage to come down and across his raisin-eyed moon-face with an almighty *klap*. But it wasn't me. *She* did it – it was her fine, fiery spirit of indignation that rose up within me like a vengeful Ouija board. *How dare you?* – that was what she was saying.

So as I lay there in the delivery room, I knew very well who was coming. I only had to get through the pain. The pain was the stranger I had to meet before I could be reunited with my fellow traveller.

At first, the drugs administered to induce labour had no effect. I walked around for a while, dragging my drip with me to get the stuff flowing through my veins. It did not feel like a great day, but a dreary day with linoleum passageways and bored patients. I sent my mother and my husband away. A nurse put a new and stronger dose of drugs into the drip bag, officiously checking the flow.

Slowly, towards afternoon, the contractions came, a sensation that is only called pain for want of a more appropriate word. The word might be 'alienation', since the body turns on itself, forcing open the pelvis, the cervix, stretching the perineum. Utter alienation. I felt no connection to anything that was happening to me in the cold loneliness of the little ante-room where they wheeled me. The nurses lived their own lives. They came in occasionally to see if I was dilated and by how much. They checked the drip. They took my blood pressure, consulting their fob watches so as to avoid eye contact. Later one came in and broke my waters to speed things up. Through it all I lay

15

there passively, waiting to become an emergency.

Now the contractions came more frequently. I had thought they would be a part of me, the way a stomach-ache is. But they were a force that operated upon my body, not from within it, as if directed by someone I could not see, someone who was working the controls and observing me through one-way glass. The antenatal classes had been, as I'd suspected, a complete waste of time. I could no more manage my breathing now than could a victim of medieval instruments of torture.

I was wheeled into the labour ward. I felt a strong urge to get up onto my knees, but the nurse said that would affect the foetal heart monitor. The waves were coming so rapidly now, looming up above me in vertiginous towers, that I was sure my little yacht would capsize. I could not say that the pain was in my abdomen or my pelvis – it pervaded every last ventricle of my being, so that I called to my husband, who had returned at last in the guise of one marooned on a cartoon desert island, 'Tell them to amputate my arms, my legs.'

Ordinary pain is a familiar thing: toothache and headache and lumbago are instantly recognisable and we hail them by their names. These familiar pains spring no surprises, and as we submit ourselves to them, we know their probable intensity and duration. But childbirth is the singular pain, the one that bursts the blood vessels in the eyes and forces bile up into the mouth. It is a pain of such magnitude that it nearly kills the woman as it brings her through the narrow, privileged passage of transfiguration. She will never be the same again, because she will be stronger – ready for the screeching siren ride to the emergency room clutching a blank-eyed child; ready for the phone call in the middle of the night; ready, indeed, for all the nights. It is a tempering pain, a pain caused by melting at high temperatures, adding an alloy and then beating the resulting metal into a shield.

I was in the midst of it when I remembered my older sister's advice on childbirth: 'I've got three words for you, Nuala: EP-I-DURAL.' I called across the machines and kidney bowls to my husband. 'Science!' I said. 'I want science!' He knew what I meant.

'Are you sure?' queried the nurse. 'It'll only be another hour or so.' Another hour? I didn't have another five minutes in me. Luckily my husband is blessed with the same strong spirit of defiance and indignation as my daughter.

'Get an anaesthetist immediately!' he insisted.

But the man would have to be summoned from across town, said the nurse. Like many choleric people, my husband welcomed opposition. Now he could point out in polysyllables exactly why it was the anaesthetist's Hippocratic duty to drive across town and render his services! Now he could have a fight! Now he could boom across the passageways and call himself 'Doctor' (as his Ph.D. rather confusingly allowed)! Now there would be a trouncing! He would take no prisoners! Tears would be shed in the linen room that evening! It was really quite satisfying to lie there and watch Rumpelstiltskin stamp his feet at someone else for a change.

The anaesthetist arrived speedily and warned me to sit absolutely still on the edge of the gurney while he injected my lower spine. He was the candy man: I would have done anything for him.

Ah, the peace, the relief. This was civilisation at its highest. Now a nurse had to tell me when I was having a contraction; I had to be told when to push, push, push.

More and more people came into the room. They spoke loudly to me and to each other. I understood, but could not feel, that birth was imminent. The nurse had already had her first sight of my daughter's head when the gynaecologist finally made his cheery appearance.

I did not feel the episiotomy. Then, for an instant, the room changed and was filled with a different kind of light – the sensation was of a lightning flash or an old-fashioned Hollywood flashbulb. 'It's a girl,' someone confirmed.

In the right-hand corner of the room, my daughter became the subject of various medical experiments before she was handed to me wrapped in a green hospital towel. She looked cross, wet, red and ugly. I felt an immense pity for her, that we had made her leave that warm, floating womb where she had been her natural age (my daughter will always be thirty-four – she is thirty-four now that she is only fourteen, and she will continue to be thirty-four when she is seventy) and forced her out into the fluorescent light of Pretoria Hospital on 10 September 1993 as a defenceless neonate.

I was stitched up, but something went wrong: the bleeding did not stop. Later that night I heard two nurses having a conversation over my nether regions. NURSE 1: 'But he told us not to phone him – he's gone away for the weekend.' NURSE 2: '*Vok* him. She's paying for his services and he can just come right back here and fix his own mistake.'

I was wheeled back under the fluorescent light in the middle of the night, having satisfactorily ruined my gynaecologist's weekend getaway.

I woke the next morning with a hunger that immediately put an end to my fifteen-year stint as a vegetarian. I could have shot and eaten an impala.

It was even more important that Beatrice should develop an appetite. We would not be released until she latched on, warned the German nurse who was in charge of torturing my nipples. She squeezed them expertly between her fingers, and my humiliation poured out in a strong white stream.

'Please latch on,' I whispered to little Beats. 'We have to get out of here.' She didn't really want to drink, and never actually took to my left breast at all, but for the sake of freedom, she tucked in. Then we went home and made our own life, with cabarets and applause and chocolates and the rhythm of the beat.

The Waiting Room

Sarah Nuttall

I first saw her legs in Port Elizabeth. But what I remember, more than her legs, is the bend in the road leading to the hospital entrance. I can picture the cement kerb, the red-striped boom, the man in his kiosk. Why is it that we can remember ordinary things and not the things we think we will never forget? These days I sometimes wonder, will I remember this, or this, or this, or none of these? What will *now* be, *then*? So I remember the tarred road winding ahead of the kiosk towards a low-slung building. And four of us sitting on a bench on the grass having a cup of tea. My mother wearing white and a silver cross. My father with his sloping smile. A.'s silence. Me in a summer dress a little tight around the waist.

The real thing was seeing her legs. Not just her legs. Legs and arms, the bones of her spine, vaulting in a fish tank. It's just that now I can't remember exactly, as exactly as I would like to remember, how they really looked then, on that computer screen. That's what I want to see again, what I want to hold on to, but can't get back to. A bit like looking at a photograph of someone, younger, and seeing that that person, precisely as he or she was then, will never again exist in this world. It's not quite that I want her back as she was then, fish in a tank, it's that she's gone already, blurred, fuzzy.

On the way in, there had been virtually nothing to talk about. Gamtoos, Kabeljous, Patensie, Uitenhage. Arum lilies pert in dishevelled *vleis*. The wide, flat, white beaches of the Indian Ocean. Fynbos seguing into farmland. My mind drifted. A friend from Wisconsin had written to say that he was staying in his mother's flat in P.E. And that living in her block now were Rwandans, Somalians, Nigerians. The wide roads of the small city. The low suburban walls that Johannesburgers would regard as breathtakingly naive.

I must have looked like any other woman coming for a scan. Which I was. Except that I came with a story. Not that any other woman doesn't have a story. We had by now moved into the waiting room, since it was time for my appointment. A puffy couch or two, floral prints on the wall. A radio playing. Plenty of light. Two people came out, her face grey and wet, his arm curved across her shoulder. Then it was my turn. I told the doctor my story, briefly. He didn't look particularly shocked. It's good to tell a story and to feel that it's part of how we all live. Just something (terrible) that happened. To feel that it is a story which might belong to someone else, another woman, but which in fact is mine.

This visit to the doctor in Port Elizabeth was all because of something that had happened six weeks before. I had become ill, though in an unspecific way. The main symptom was a heavy tiredness. I slept and slept. And when I woke I watched the trees outside my bedroom window, following the shapes of the branches in such detail that it was as if I myself was drawing them. On the third day I dragged myself to the early morning session at my gynaecologist's rooms. As usual, the waiting room was full – women mostly, dressed for work, queuing early to be tested in some way, for something. On the walls, spiky abstracts in turquoise, purple and grey. A radio playing. All the best magazines taken. Finally it was my turn. The gynaecologist's assistant had already done a blood test. I had had some spotting – the first time I hadn't had a proper period (apart from when I was pregnant before). Was it a fibroid? Was I becoming too thin? Now the little white plastic box with its window was given to me. The two lines formed a blood-red cross. 'Four weeks,' the doctor said. 'And everything looks fine.' Last time a doctor told me things would be fine it had been a lie and he knew it. But now, as I looked at the late November clouds through the car window, I began to believe this other man, this other doctor. But I pretended to myself that I didn't.

A week later we went on holiday to Cape Town. To my family home. We hired a small red car and wound our way around the mountain, to Clarke's Bookshop and on to Mouille

Point. I found another waiting room. Each week for the next three weeks I went there. A. would surround himself with the newspaper. I would go through the door. It was too much for us both to go, we had to keep one of us in reserve. So each week I went through the door on my own, changed into a blue nightgown in a tiny room and sat on a bed waiting for the doctor to do a scan. Then I dressed and walked back down the corridor. A.'s face met mine as he looked for a sign that there was no disaster yet. That a loss had been averted. For now. The newspaper lay crumpled on the chair.

In Port Elizabeth, it was time to go through for the scan. My mother was with me. The wet jelly, the probe on my tummy and, suddenly, the moving image on the screen. Fishy in her fish tank. At ten weeks, a baby has hands with fingers and feet with toes that it can move. Outside the glass doors of the small side room where we were, a peacock fussed in the scrubby dust. My mother had never seen such a thing, a ten-week-old human form. Afterwards, I couldn't stop talking. I talked all the way to Woolworths where I bought the silliest things, things that I never eat anyway. I can't remember anything that we saw on the drive back down to the coast, because everyone in the car was talking. I was listening to the talking.

$\bigcirc$

When my first baby, Mia Fabienne, was born, I was lying in the theatre waiting when my doctor came in and said, 'Why do you look so nervous? It will be fine.' I had last seen him at six thirty that evening when he had said that we would need to do an emergency Caesarean and that he would see me at seven p.m. An hour and a half ago. I didn't feel anything as they made the incision. I looked up at A.'s face. In ten minutes or so I heard a baby cry. The clock on the wall said ten past eight. The baby was taken over to a table at the side. I strained my head to see. A doctor was using what looked like bellows. 'Is the baby all right?' I asked into the ceiling of the theatre. 'She's just a bit lazy,' said the anaesthetist. I asked again. 'She's fine,' my doctor said. I was wheeled out of the theatre. And parked in a side room. After a few minutes my doctor came in. He was already showered and dressed in his brown leather jacket. I looked at him. 'Is the baby all right?' I said. 'Your baby's fine,' he answered. 'But anyway, it's over to the paediatrician now.' He left. A nurse wheeled me out of the theatre area towards the lifts.

I saw my mother and father sitting in two white plastic chairs outside the lift. My mother stood up and came towards me. 'I don't know where my baby is,' I said to her. 'It took so long,' she said. The lift closed behind me.

○

Now, in my second pregnancy, in the months of February to June, we made weekly trips from my office at Wits to Linkwood Clinic with its lakes and trees. The feel of that time is Louis Botha Avenue. Again it is the road that I see. Psychologists would say that my unconscious was insisting I was on a journey. I prefer the more literal-minded idea of the road itself. At the bottom end of Hillbrow the flatlands of Groot Drakenstein, Kings Langley and Royal Crescent, Africans from both here and other places leaning over the balconies, hanging washing, watching, listening, sitting. Then on the left The Wilds and Avenue Mansions, and taxis darting, lumbering, screeching across the top of Houghton. Further on, around the Yeoville bend, is Ahmed's Café, Sanaz Butchery and Braai, Christian Pentecostal International and the Enlightened Security Head Office. And on the last stretch before the turn-off to Linkwood Hospital, the Victory Theatre, Radium Beerhall, Tombstone Showroom, Spread the Word Ministry and Miracle Centre, the Kosher B&B and Yeshiva Cottage. On the other side of the hill, Roberts Road and Blenheim Street, Vladislavić territory. Once or twice, when I am in Kensington, I drive down Bleinheim Street, just to feel the overlay of Vladislavić's writing, to inhabit a written city. To see the 'spare poetry' of the city's landmarks from the ridge and to have his words float in on the air: 'This is our climate. We have grown up in this air, this light, we grasp it on the skin, where it grasps us.' A city which so often alienates us who live in it, seems strange to us, but which yields up moments in which 'we will never be closer to who we are than this'.[1]

In May sometime, when I was feeling particularly tired, my doctor gave me the name of a person who does massages for pregnant women. I liked going to her. She herself had no children, so she helped women who were going to give birth. She always put the blind down in the room where she worked, and I always asked her to put it up again, so I could see the trees and the sunlight slanting into the room. She would mention that the neighbours might be able to see in, and I would say, let's take a chance. One time, she suggested that we use visualisation. OK, I said, and so she began. She wanted me to visualise the scene of my last birth, in the theatre, to flood that scene with light and to replace what happened there with what I would have wanted to happen. To see it, go right into it, and to replace it. Is it possible to flee from a scene when one is lying flat on one's back? To come to a screeching halt, to turn around and run for one's life? I cannot do that, I said to her. I must have been breathing very fast. OK, she said. Let's go somewhere else. Or I could just rub your back?

○

That evening, once I had come out of the theatre and seen my mother at the lifts, I was wheeled along another corridor. Into the ICU. My mother reappeared. I was shown a baby in a glass box with wire cords all over her. She was really big. She was very beautiful. I couldn't touch her. I looked. She's very white, I said. No one answered. I was wheeled out again, into a small room with a single bed. I felt my way into a deep sleep. Something shocking had happened.

In the morning I was wheeled back into the ICU. She lay in a different bed now, in a room on her own, and the lid was off.

---

1 Ivan Vladislavić, *Portrait with Keys: The City of Johannesburg Unlocked.* Cape Town: Umuzi, 2006.

I sat with her and looked at her. It was as if she wasn't mine. I couldn't believe that she had come out of me. She must have been four kilograms. Her legs and arms were strong and she had the loveliest lips. Her face was not puckered like some babies. It was round and smooth and less white than it was the night before. But she wasn't mine. So this is what childbirth is like. I was amazed by her. But how could I love her when I couldn't touch her? I wrapped my summer dressing gown around me more closely.

In the evening, my brother, a paediatrician from Cape Town, arrived. My mother said to go with him to show him my baby. No, I said. A. went with him instead. My brother said that she was beautiful and also that the first twenty-four hours are crucial in determining a baby's chances. During the night hours A. and I tried to sleep, but A. had to half lie in a chair alongside the bed. When my brother came back the next day in the late morning, he was terribly sick. He was pale, and he could hardly stand up. His body looked as if it would fold beneath him. As if he was swaying on a boat at sea, struggling to hold on to an invisible rail. We sat in the café downstairs. My parents didn't seem to realise how sick he was. I thought it was perhaps because he realised Mia wasn't going to be all right, that he was sick with what he knew but couldn't say to me. That morning a psychologist had been sent to see me at eight a.m. 'You shouldn't worry,' he said, perched on the end of my bed while I struggled to wake. 'We've had over fifty cases of asphyxia in this hospital and the babies are always all right in the end.' It's not asphyxia, I could have said. Even though no one had told me what it was. 'Shame, such a beautiful baby,' the paediatrician had said. 'But she's a very, very sick girl, you know.' The psychologist must have known by the way I looked at him that I wanted him to leave.

○

Now, in my second pregnancy, it was late June and I was starting to feel that there might be something that we weren't picking up. That at the last minute there would be something that we

24

had missed. That we might still lose her. I went to Linkwood to ask for a foetal monitor to be strapped to my tummy. I lay there listening to her heartbeat, amplified across the room.

○

On the sixth day after Mia's birth I was still there. In the evening, around nine, the paediatrician came in. 'What time is the CAT scan tomorrow?' I asked him. 'We're not going to do a CAT scan,' he said. That's odd, I thought. I had planned to go along with her. That night I went home and lay in my own bed. Suddenly I knew. For myself. It was over. She was going to die. After the doctor left, I had said to the nurse, 'Why do you think they aren't going to do a brain scan?' 'Because they already know what they need to know,' she'd said. In bed I recalled that, but it was really the way the paediatrician had said 'such a beautiful baby' instead of something else that made me know in the muscles and ventricles of my heart that it was over.

A meeting had been set for ten the next morning. It was to be the paediatrician, my parents, A. and me. In a small room adjacent to the ICU. We waited. The paediatrician was late, and a call came through to say he was still in theatre. I lay with my head next to Mia, and I spread my hair on her chest. We were the closest we had ever been. Waiting for him was like waiting for nothing. It was only her and me. When he came I stood up. He signalled for us to proceed to the room at the end. The others started off. I stopped him. 'Don't hurt them,' I said. He looked at me and I could see that he knew then that I knew. I refused to leave the small room where Mia Fabienne lay. A. came back. My parents had gone into the room. 'I don't want you to hurt them,' I said. The paediatrician looked at me. I took A. in my arms and held him tightly. The paediatrician said: 'Your child has third-degree damage. She lost too much oxygen. She cannot survive.'

○

At Linkwood, lying there with the foetal monitor on, I knew it couldn't happen again. But I still couldn't get away, at least not fully, from the only birth story I had known. I was repeating it, replaying it, and at the same time trying to set it right. I knew I was different from how I had been then, an altered person. But still, I couldn't quite separate from that other, earlier self, the one that had never had a baby before. For the second time in a week, I lay in the room listening. To her. Watching the printout of her heart. Feeling the feeling of two hearts in one body. Waiting for Friday. Thirty-eight weeks. The day of the Caesarean.

○

I carried on holding A. He held me. We sat like that in the plastic chair. The paediatrician went to tell my parents. After a while, I got up and walked out of the ICU. I took the stairs and walked out of the hospital. I found a place where some water was falling, near the entrance, and I sat down next to the water, in the sun. If the eternal emptiness of shock could have a texture, be a substance, that was what I was now made of. No tears. Only the water falling, and the sun, and me.

○

On Wednesday we drove through the dead of night. That afternoon I had said to her, 'You're going to be born on Friday, but whenever you want to come, just come.' She woke me with her decision around midnight. As we drove, she did the nicest thing. She kicked me a bit. She wriggled. I knew she was there. Still, I gripped the door handle in the car and said nothing. Heading towards a cut. A deep incision. After that, I could see nothing. Was it really possible that they would pull a baby out of me – and give her to me? That I would see her? That she would be all right?

They must have given me a light sedative. When they put her next to me, her head next to mine, I said, 'Don't you want to check her?' I remember the paediatrician saying, in her light Croatian accent, 'If I thought there was anything wrong, I would have taken her to check.' Do you want to breastfeed her? someone else asked me. I stared at her. It was as if I was watching from a very long way away. I remembered A.'s gasp when she came out, with her eyes open. They wheeled me back upstairs. Next to me I had a small bundle. I couldn't stop shaking. I shook for almost two hours. 'Why am I shaking?' I asked. 'It sometimes happens,' said the midwife. I shook so much that the bed rattled. It was two thirty a.m. I held her all night. I wanted to sleep but I wouldn't let myself. I checked her breathing every five minutes. If I sleep, I said to myself, I might lose her. She might stop breathing.

Twenty-four hours later I fell asleep for a while. When I woke she was still there.

○

In the evenings we have a bath together. She sits in the triangle I make with my legs. She plays with her frogs and ducks, and inspects the lemon tree outside the window. These days she rubs her hand on the soap and swishes it on her chest, washing herself, imitating me. We play and play, and when we are finished we line up the frogs and the ducks on the edge of the bath, blow out the candle – and leave everything in place for tomorrow night.

Making Finn

Susan Newham and Roxi Blake

'I'm pregnant!' said Susan. 'It wasn't me,' I joked, but at the same time wished it had been.

Then I cried. I was blown away.

When the day came, Susan called me at work to say she thought she was in labour. I packed my bag but didn't shut down my computer, because I was sure I'd be back in an hour or two. I never did make it back to work that day – or for the next ten days, in fact.

Our baby boy was born at 7:20 the following morning. Susan's strength through the raw and unforgiving labour deepened my love and respect for her. And witnessing the miracle of our son's birth, I knew this was something I wanted to do myself one day.

We named our baby Finn. He is an embodiment of our love and determination, the most precious gift I have ever received.

Before our baby was conceived, half his genetic make-up in the form of six vials of semen was flown in a nitrogen vapour tank from San Francisco to New York to Paris to Johannesburg and then to Cape Town, where I had been waiting for some time. Two months previously, on a quest to find out whether it was even possible to fly semen from a sperm bank in the States to South Africa, I had been given the number of the South African Customs helpline. On hearing my query, the young man on the other end of the phone went silent. After a short pause he gathered himself enough to say, 'But can't you find that kind of stuff in South Africa?' I assured the man that my request was as surprising to me as it was to him.

As a little girl, my favourite doll was a 'First Love' called Jenny, who went everywhere with me. Every day, when I got home from school I would rush over to pick Jenny up from my bed, and would spend the rest of the day wandering around with her attached to my hip. In the early evenings I would stand on tiptoe and kiss the doorframe, pretending it was my make-believe husband, Stephen, returning from work. I never doubted that this fantasy family would one day become a reality.

Years later, nearing thirty and very much single, I found myself in crisis. With a string of failed relationships with men behind me, I had to face something that I had been fighting internally since my teens: the fear that I might be gay. I resolved with some trepidation to embrace my feelings, hoping that this would provide clarity.

Clarification arrived in the form of a petite but fiery woman with glossy black hair and enormous brown eyes who shared my sense of humour and passion for life. She also shared my dream of having a family. The big question was, how would the two of us make a baby?

I became consumed by this dilemma and – as I often do during times of turmoil – I turned to Google. One morning, sitting at my desk at work, I typed in the words 'artificial insemination south africa'. I discovered that all manner of animals, including elephants, are inseminated artificially in our glorious game parks. I also discovered the website of a reputable fertility clinic that offered to inseminate women who, for whatever reason, did not have access to fertile, healthy sperm.

Two weeks later my partner, Roxi, and I walked hand in hand up the clinic stairs. My heart thumped from nervousness, but also from excitement – as if, somehow, a quick trip to the fertility clinic was all it would take to get me pregnant and start the family we so wished for. We'd agreed that I would try first because I had fewer years of fertility left than Roxi did.

And yet the mild-mannered doctor who explained the available conception options left me feeling confused and doubtful. We learnt that in South Africa insemination with sperm from an anonymous donor meant that our child would know nothing about one half of his biological roots, other than a third of a page of information supplied by the clinic – hair, eye and skin colour; height and weight; and a brief summary written by the donor describing himself. There were only twelve donors to choose from.

That evening, Roxi and I sat staring at the twelve pieces of paper bearing each donor's description. We were mute. Since there was no logical way to make this kind of decision, we eventually hit on a plan to hide the donors' physical data and read only their personal descriptions. The man we liked best described himself as having a great sense of humour and zest for life. He turned out to be a six-foot-tall African man who resembled neither of us. We decided to do it the other way round and read the physical specs first. We thought the Indian man, with eyes and skin the colour of Roxi's, sounded striking, but his description didn't resonate with either of us. He was introverted and liked spending time alone. I feared he might be a serial killer.

The exercise sent me reeling. The huge significance of what we were about to do paralysed me. I suddenly had severe doubts that I could go through with this and began to wonder if a known donor would be a better option. I decided to base my decision on what would be best for the well-being of the child and what would be best for the well-being of our relationship. I hoped that these would not prove to be two different scenarios.

It was only six months later, after hours of research, discussion and consultation with medical professionals, lawyers and psychologists, that we came to a decision we both felt comfortable with. We decided that we would not use a known donor because of issues I feared would later complicate our lives. From the research I had done, I knew that there could be possible abandonment issues for the child if the donor was not an active part of our baby's life. If he did become very involved, there were potential legal complications – we could get into custody battles and he would be recognised by law as a more rightful parent than Roxi. We feared that introducing a third party would dilute our family unit and create uneasy dynamics.

But deciding on an anonymous donor also seemed fraught with complications. First, I had to come to terms with my own sense of loss at not being able to give my baby a father. I also worried that our child might be haunted by not knowing half his biology. Again I turned to Google for comfort. I discovered a number of sperm banks in the United States that offered identity-release donors. These were men who donated sperm on condition that if their offspring wanted to make contact with them once they turned eighteen, they could. This suddenly seemed like a viable option – a way to protect our family and allow for the possibility of our child learning about his genetic inheritance.

I e-mailed eight sperm banks to find out if they were prepared to sell and ship their goods to South Africa. Three responded in the affirmative. They each offered long lists of donor options with the possibility of purchasing additional information, which included ten-page donor descriptions, staff impression reports and extensive medical backgrounds of each donor and his extended family. One bank even offered the option of hearing the donors' voices. I spent days with my headphones plugged into my computer so that I could listen to donors from a sperm bank in Virginia holding forth on topics as varied as the weather and what they thought of President Bush. They all sounded, well, very American.

I became immersed in donor land, accessing information on hundreds of men. All were fertile, all were HIV-negative and many sounded downright peculiar. There was a donor who'd accidentally shot himself while cleaning his gun and survived. Another described himself as driving his parents to near nervous breakdown because he'd been so hyperactive as a child. There were a few whose families were rife with addiction disorders, others with serious mental illness. To be fair, my own family tree was not entirely untainted, but unlike the donor I was a given, and didn't have to analyse the possible influence of my great-aunt's penchant for shoplifting and over-the-counter painkillers.

Even with all this information, it was impossible to make a decision. We finally decided that we'd stick to basic genetics and go for someone who looked like a combination of both of us in case Roxi wanted to become pregnant one day with the same donor. We took up an offer of a photo match and sent off photographs of ourselves to the bank not situated in redneck territory. The fact that Roxi and I look nothing alike, being of different races and entirely different colouring, couldn't have made it any easier for the people trying to match our profiles. But they came back promptly with four donors they believed would meet our standards. We chose the one who seemed least likely to produce offspring that displayed psychopathic tendencies. And if the staff report was to be believed, he also sounded intelligent, handsome and caring. My mother, in particular, liked the sound of him – so much so, I worried she might orchestrate a meeting with him even before our child got the opportunity.

The relief of having finally made a decision left Roxi and me feeling bouncy with excitement. It felt like the difficult part was over. However, getting the goods into South Africa proved a logistical challenge, entailing far too much contact with the Department of Health as we prodded them into issuing us with an ominous-sounding Import Permit for Biological Substances. And, of course, there was dealing with Customs. The man on the other end of the Customs helpline was baffled by our request. What were they to tax the sperm under? What happened if the goods were held up at Customs and thawed? The nitrogen tank could keep its contents frozen for up to two weeks, but the flying time alone could take easily as long as a week.

Eventually we employed a freight-shipping company to take over. They had contacts at Customs and could possibly help speed the process along. However, the small, weathered man assigned to our case, who spent his days primarily coordinating the import of textiles, was sceptical about our venture. 'I imported horse semen once,' he commented while shaking my hand in introduction. 'Things went horribly wrong when Customs left it lying in a back room for five days. They had to trash the whole batch.' This was not reassuring. Our whole batch, which included six vials of sperm, was not the cheapest purchase we'd ever made. Nevertheless we had done everything we could to ensure safe passage, and all we could really do was wait.

Early one Saturday morning, after many long days, our faithful freight man called to tell me he had the goods. An hour later he arrived outside the house in a silver BMW, and delivered the large grey plastic bin that contained the stainless-steel nitrogen tank and vials of precious 'biological substance'. Despite the fact that the clinic would only be open on Monday morning and we'd have to hang on to our precious container until then, Rox and I were jubilant. We spent the weekend staring at the container which we placed on the floor at the foot of our bed. 'It's Daddy,' I whispered to Roxi.

It felt strange to have gone through so much just to get to the stage where many people start the process . . . falling pregnant. I feared we might still have a long way to go. At nearly thirty-five I didn't feel quite as fertile as I once did.

For our first try, Roxi and I spent weeks preparing for the big day. Waiting to learn whether or not I was pregnant felt endless, and finally discovering that I wasn't was devastating. I resolved to be more fatalistic the second time around. On this attempt the insemination was scheduled for ten a.m. on Christmas Eve. We squeezed it in between some last-minute Christmas shopping and preparing for a Christmas Eve dinner party for twelve. Luckily, insemination is a quick and painless process and it took all of twenty-six seconds. Once completed, I continued lying on the doctor's bed for another five minutes with Rox at my side. 'Swim, little fishies, swim,' she encouraged. Afterwards, driving to the mall, I lay in the passenger seat with my legs hoisted up on the dashboard, listening to Sarah Brightman. Although the doctor had assured us that even standing on one's head was probably futile, I did have the distinct feeling, lying in the hot car trying to sing along to the opera, that this was it.

Two weeks later, feeling bloated and disappointingly premenstrual, I bought a home pregnancy test, resolving to take it first thing on the Sunday morning. That Saturday night I dreamt that it turned out positive. The following morning Roxi followed me, yawning, into the bathroom, where I nervously did the test. We stared at the white stick as a second pink line slowly began emerging next to the test strip. It had worked! I beamed with relief and excitement and pride. Roxi cried. We hugged. I called my mother, who also cried. For far longer than most of her friends, she'd secretly wished to be a grandmother.

The long months of pregnancy were a volatile journey of morning sickness, exhaustion, excited anticipation and alarm at growing so enormous so quickly. By the end of the nine months, I was more than ready for the birth.

The first signs came very early one Friday morning in September, although it was only much later that evening that the labour pains began. Because my gynaecologist had left the country that morning to visit her mother in Sweden, I was left in the hands of one of the night staff. She insisted that my requests for an epidural were too early, as I was not dilated enough, and Roxi and I were left alone in a private hospital room.

As it turned out, I dilated from one to nine centimetres in only five hours. I spent these hours without a nurse in attendance, pacing the small, stifling room in a desperate attempt to escape the pain. Although Roxi and I did not speak much during this time, every now and again she would tenderly stroke my hair and whisper, 'You're such a strong girl.' I would reply, 'Thank you for being here.' Little else needed to be said.

The epidural finally arrived half an hour before I began pushing, and with it came the most blissful relief. An hour later our little boy was born. I was transfixed by the expression on Roxi's face as she whispered, 'You're finally here.'

Today, as I hold our six-month-old son in my arms, I am still incredulous. Forging new paths without the maps of those who've gone before has made my life more difficult, yet more wondrous, than I could ever have dreamt as a little girl.

Dear Onke

Kholeka Sigenu

I have had premonitions all my life. My mother says that I was born in *isingxobo*[1] and according to the old wives' tale this meant that I would be lucky and naturally protected throughout my life. Well, I believe her.

On 2 September 1977, your father and I were driving from Blikana village to Makhulu and Tatomkhulu in Herschel, where we had arranged to spend the weekend. On the way we had to pass Umlamli Hospital. I had a strong feeling that I was close to giving birth, even though I was just entering the seventh month of pregnancy. I wanted to ask your father to leave me at the hospital, but I didn't say anything. Later we also passed Sterkspruit Hospital, but still I kept quiet about my premonition.

That night, at Makhulu and Tatomkhulu's house, my waters broke suddenly. I did not know what was happening. I thought it was urine, that I was wetting the bed, and I was very embarrassed. There were no prenatal classes in our villages. We were kept in the dark. Everything about childbirth was shrouded in secrecy, even though we went to Umlamli Hospital monthly for check-ups.

Tata went to tell Makhulu that I was passing water and that it would not stop. I was standing on a big towel next to my bed by this time. Luckily a friend who was a trained nurse was also visiting for the weekend. She realised that I was in labour and ordered Tata to drive me to Umlamli Hospital immediately.

When we arrived at the hospital, I was told that I was very close to giving birth. I was given a bed in the labour ward. However, your birth did not take place that night, and miraculously I felt no labour pains either. This gave me an opportunity to quench

1 'A caul'.

my curiosity about the two other women in the ward. The younger one was a sixteen-year-old, I learnt later. The older woman was, in my estimation, between fifty and sixty. She had no idea when she was born. At over twenty-nine, I was somewhere between them.

As it happened, the youngest gave birth first, easily and quietly, with the help of only one nurse. Then she passed out with exhaustion. The nurse explained that the young ones gave the least problems. Seeing that teenager give birth with such ease made me confident that it would be easy for me too. The older lady was next, and her behaviour was quite the opposite. She screamed and shouted until several nurses came to help. She was oblivious when they scolded her; she just yelled her way through the pain and gave birth to a bouncing baby. As soon as she heard the baby cry she smiled, then laughed outright when it was given to her to hold.

It left me wondering what it would be like when my turn came.

The morning nurse had given me some castor oil without explaining that she was inducing birth. It was only much later that I understood what she had done. I thought at the time that I was being given a purgative. Therefore, when my turn came, I thought the purgative was beginning to work. The two ladies who had already given birth said that I should not stand up, but ring a bell for the nurse. Although I questioned why I should call a nurse when I simply wanted to obey the call of nature, I did as they said.

By the time she arrived I was feeling very uncomfortable and beginning to whine. Then somebody went to call the doctor. Now let me tell you about Notyiphana.[2] (That is what the doctor was called because she had a lean body.) Every patient at Umlamli, a Roman Catholic mission hospital, loved and respected her. She was the only doctor at the hospital then, so it was like *her* hospital. She liked me very much because I, too, had a very small build and was not a local. Once she told a hefty

---

2 The name means 'small chicken'.

nurse who had been nasty to me, 'Kholeka is not an *intombi*;[3] she is married.' I shall tell you more about that nurse later. Once Notyiphana told me, 'I am the only doctor who is doubly qualified. I wrote my Ph.D. in Germany and I wrote another one when I arrived in *Sous Africa*.' She taught me everything about raising a child, because she knew that my mother lived far away in Queenstown. She always looked very busy, but she made a point of conversing with me whenever I went to the hospital for check-ups. Mostly we talked about our parents. It made me feel special.

Notyiphana arrived just as the pain was becoming unbearable. At last you, my son, were born. You made a cat-like noise. Then I felt intense pain and yelled, 'Another baby is coming!' To my astonishment, Notyiphana delivered your twin. Although it might seem absurd in these days of information, I had not known that I was carrying twins. Nor could I have known their gender. It was therefore amazing to discover that I had given birth to a beautiful son and daughter at the same time.

A few minutes later, again I shouted, 'Another baby is coming!' The good doctor came back and said, 'No child is coming. I should know, I'm the doctor.' She must have been very tired and did not catch the joke. She is the best doctor Umlamli could ever have had. She got rid of the afterbirth, for that is just what it was.

The only inkling I had had that I might be carrying twins was during an X-ray scan early in my pregnancy. I had consulted a private doctor because I was experiencing several uncomfortable symptoms. When the doctor showed me that the baby was in a breech position, I thought I saw two embryos. However, he said nothing and I kept this to myself.

The pure joy I felt when you were born was short-lived. Your sister had been exposed to radiation from the X-ray, and because of this she developed a second fontanelle on the stomach. She therefore passed away three days later. I regretted so deeply that I had consulted a doctor. I did not know about

3 'A girl'.

the danger of having an X-ray when pregnant. I know now how very expensive ignorance is. Had I known what I know today about scans, I would never have agreed to an X-ray.

I was very sad to lose my lovely baby girl, but I was left with you, Onke, a precious boy. My feelings were so confused. I mourned your twin who had passed away and at the same time I rejoiced, for I still had a baby. I decided not to mourn for too long and instead prayed for you to survive. This was a scary situation, as your sister, at 1.2 kilograms, had looked healthier than you. You weighed only 1 kilogram.

You were my tiny miracle. You were so small; I could carry you in my two open hands. I was afraid of closing my hands as I feared I might crush your bones. Your feet were as small as my little finger. You were placed in an incubator – your second womb, as I called it.

Our stay in the hospital was quite an adventure. I was taught how to express milk and tube-feed you. One night, the hefty nurse was on duty. I kept expressing and leaving milk for you to be tube-fed, but at the next feed I would find the last milk still standing where I had put it. I questioned the nurse, explaining that I had been taught the skill of expressing milk for you, but she would not allow me to use my breast milk to feed you. She was rude. My child! I hope I will never, ever be as unhappy as I was that day. I stayed in the bathroom and cried my heart out. Fortunately the matron resolved the matter and a new, kind sister replaced the hefty nurse. She was very encouraging. She taught me how to knit you lovely clothes. She would take you out of the incubator and wrap you in baby blankets so that I could hold you. Then she would put two cushions on my lap before letting me teach you how to feed from my breasts.

Do you want to know my feelings? I was the proudest mother on earth. I was ecstatic. There was warmth in my heart. After feeding you, I would go to the bathroom and sing.

Your father was obviously also very proud. He visited us at the hospital every evening. He brought the baby hamper I had ordered the day after you were born. Coincidentally, it had two of everything, as if it were known that I had had twins.

You would sense his presence and throw your eyes back as if to look at him. If you happened to cry in the incubator, you would wave your hands in the air and the nurses, who seemed to rejoice with us at our miracle, would say, 'He will be a choir conductor like his mother.' They also predicted that you would be a clever child, saying that you had decided to be born early because you were curious. My stay at the hospital was made bearable by such remarks.

There was a small Roman Catholic chapel in the hospital yard, where I made it a habit to go and pray for everything good for you, my son. Some who had been there when you were born would tease me, 'Imagine, Kholeka, giving us such a hard time when birthing, only to give birth to a "mouse".'

One day there was a fearsome thunderstorm. The thunder and lightning were so bad that even I, who am usually unafraid of storms, was concerned. Suddenly all the mothers with children in incubators were sent for. The lightning had damaged the power supply for the incubators, and there was no back-up generator. Our babies were wrapped in blankets and placed in tiny cots. They were never returned to the incubators again. I breast-fed you, my baby, until my backbone ached. I looked forward to the day when you would weigh at least two kilograms, and we could go home.

In the meantime, nurse Mary, the kind one, was making a beautiful outfit with her knitting needles. In reply to my question whether you could ever catch up with your peers, she said: 'I am making this outfit for his christening. By the time he is christened, he will fit into these clothes.' Unbelievable as it was, it was music to my ears. Truly, it happened just as she said.

I watched you grow as in a womb. Over the three months that you were in the incubator I was able to observe your metamorphosis – from a pitch-black, skinny baby to a plump and very handsome, light-complexioned boy. You were as hairy as Esau at birth, but by the time you were 'born again' you looked like all newborns, only sweeter, as you were not wrinkled like most newborn babies. I marvelled at all the changes. At last you had reached an acceptable 'birth weight' and we were able to go home. I take 3 September as your birthday, yet I will never forget the date of your second birth, 11 December, when we left the hospital.

The day you arrived at home was wondrous. Makhulu could not believe her eyes. She kept saying, 'A baby in this home after sixteen years?' Everybody marvelled at how mature your face looked for a baby your age and yet how tiny you were compared to newborns. When you looked drowsy, I wondered where to make your bed. One visitor suggested: 'Put him in a shoebox.'

Another visitor commented, 'What a beautiful girl you've got there.' When I replied that you were a boy, she said, '*Uyak'tshata phi*?'[4] It was unbelievable to her that such a good-looking baby could be a boy. Where would he find a match in marriage? You were handsome indeed.

It is surprising how quickly you grew after that, considering that you did not want to breast-feed. You were a quiet child and yet very temperamental. You were also observant and wanted your signature on everything you saw – paper, soil, stones. In fact, one day you saw your father signing school reports (he was a school principal) and you decided to sit quietly next to him and follow suit. We knew then that you were destined for success.

You were special in a number of ways. You were not only my first-born, but also a son, something very important in our culture. Moreover, you were a twin as well as a premature baby.

The fact that you were a twin brought both happiness and heartache for me. The birth of twins is shrouded in superstition. The good superstition is that the mother of twins brings good luck and wealth to the home. So, if there are hailstones, the mother of twins is asked to take a stone or a broom and throw it away, crying '*Embo*!', and the storm ceases. If there are pumpkin plants in the garden, the mother of twins is asked to walk over them. The result is that the family will reap plenty during the reaping season.

---

4 'Where will he get married?'

But I was very anxious about another superstition called *ukuretla*. According to some people in Herschel, the use of body parts to make *muti*[5] that bestows wealth is rife. The body parts of a twin are allegedly twice as enriching, since twins are seen as good luck. The parts are supposedly taken when the person is still alive, and he or she is left to die later. The belief is that if you put body parts from a twin among the seeds while you are planting, you will reap a very rich harvest. That was my real fear for you as you grew up. I watched you like a hawk.

For us Africans the naming of a child is a matter of great importance. We name our children after an event, or we give a prophetic name, one that we hope the child will live up to. So when you were born, almost everyone wanted to give you a name. You ended up having three.

Because you were born at Umlamli Hospital, Tatomkhulu named you *Mlamli*. I voiced my concern that I had had a cousin by that name and he had turned out to be a gangster. So I refused that name for you, my child, and thus he called you *Lamla*, which means 'peacemaker'. I am married into the Hlubi tribe, whose custom is to name especially the first son with the name given to his mother by her in-laws as a sign of accepting her into her new home (just like a newborn daughter). My married name is *No-Onke* (why they named me that is another story). So you naturally inherited the name *Onke*. And then I named you *Thando*[6] because you were born at the height of your parents' love. Your three names make up a lovely sentence: *Lamla Onke (amaTolo ngo) Thando*.[7] How prophetic names sometimes turn out to be!

---

5 'Medication'.
6 'Love'.
7 Loosely translated, this means 'Dish justice/peace to the Tolo clan peacefully/lovingly.'

I Gave My Love a Cherry

Vanessa September & Albie Sachs

Once a year, on Boxing Day, my family used to set off with great excitement, by train, for Kalk Bay beach. Except that the little strip of sand couldn't really be called a beach. With almost everybody from the Cape Flats there at the same time, one could barely see the sand! On the journey there, I used to look out of the train window. Along the suburban railway line were big houses in wide streets, with large, leafy gardens. We lived in a small council house, with one bedroom for all eight children. The community centre up the road was the only place to go for a bit of relief. I promised myself that one day I would build houses like the ones I saw every year from the train window for people like *us*. I would be an architect.

At the age of sixteen I left school to help support my family. After doing administrative work for fourteen years, in shops, banks and other places, I applied to the University of Cape Town to study architecture, only to be turned down because I didn't have a matric. I registered at a college as soon as I could. At sixteen and seventeen, the students were nearly half my age!

It was during the previous year, just before my thirtieth birthday, that I met Albie. He supported my dream of studying architecture and encouraged me with my studies. At the end of my matric year, he asked if I was going to the matric dance. I couldn't tell him that my reluctance to attend was because he was older than the school principal! But he encouraged me to have the full 'matric experience'. On the evening of the dance he stood in line with me to have our picture taken and we opened the dance floor. Someone had the sensitivity to seat us at a table with the teachers, some of whom were my age.

At that time we weren't so sure that we'd be together for the long haul, let alone have a baby together. Albie wasn't even convinced that he wanted to have a relationship with a woman thirty-one years his junior. I, too, had doubts, but mostly I am guided by my emotions, and I wasn't budging. I wanted to see if the Albie Sachs I'd fallen in love with when I read *Soft Vengeance of a Freedom Fighter* was still present in the man I'd just got to know.

Albie and I come from different sides of the railway line, literally and figuratively, thanks to apartheid planning. You couldn't find two people more different from each other in terms of culture and background and life's work. And yet, and yet. I found in Albie a warm, kind, loving and affectionate person. I guess he found me warm and kind and loving too!

Our age difference didn't worry me. I'll catch up, I thought. Albie, on the other hand, could imagine us having ten wonderful years together. After that he wanted me to be free. I would be in the prime of my life when he would be preparing to wind down. Ten wonderful years, he thought. Except, of course, life doesn't work that way. You don't suddenly stop loving someone after ten years of being together.

My family was tickled pink by the idea of me dating a judge! My mother simply told Albie, 'I'm not surprised. Vanessa can do anything she decides on in life.' My family embraced Albie as warmly as he embraced them. Albie's mom knew me only by voice and touch; she had lost her sight by then. Still, we became very close in the two years before she died at ninety-three.

In the early part of our relationship, whenever family or friends brought up the subject of children, I used to say that I'd raised my three younger sisters and helped to bring up some of their children; I'd 'been there and done that' with child raising. It wasn't important that I have my own. I couldn't have been more mistaken! By the time I graduated in 2003, Albie and I had been together for nine years. Our lives were so strongly connected that having a baby together seemed a perfectly natural development.

I was thirty-eight and Albie was sixty-nine when I decided that if I wasn't pregnant by my fortieth birthday, I would visit a specialist. The month of my fortieth, we were on a two-week, eight-city speaking tour across the United States, talking about democracy and transformation in South Africa through our personal experiences. It was a whirlwind tour that was going to end in Los Angeles on the eve of my birthday. I didn't want to be on the long flight home on this special occasion, so Albie proposed a short holiday somewhere. Did I want to go to Las Vegas? Yes! I was so excited that he couldn't bring himself to say, 'It was a joke! It was a *joke!*' So off to Vegas we went.

I loved Vegas. Albie loathed it. We didn't marry, we didn't gamble – but as it turned out, we hit the jackpot on my fortieth birthday! Two weeks after arriving home, I bought a few do-it-yourself pregnancy tests. Together we sat on the bed and watched the test move from neutral . . . to positive!

We were joyous and wanted to tell our friends and family immediately. But, with 111 years between us, we thought it best to wait. We did the first scan when our little bean was only five millimetres long and six weeks into gestation. The twelve-week tests determined that all was well. We felt that there was no need to have an amniocentesis.

Usually people marry, have children and grow old together. That's the sequence. But we were very happy together in our life partnership and thought it worked particularly well precisely because we were *not* tied by legal bonds. We loved and respected each other and were quite content to remain in this unattached attachment. But with a baby coming, we decided that we would like to make a more formal commitment. The venue was to be the Constitutional Court. Chief Justice Pius Langa had to apply to be acting magistrate in order to marry us. The Constitutional Court Choir practised a new song for the marriage ceremony. A small circle of friends and family attended what was an intimate and emotional occasion. (I looked very large in my Marianne Fassler wedding dress!)

After nine uncomplicated months of antenatal classes and regular visits to Dr Somaya Ebrahim, our gynaecologist, and Phindi Mashini, our midwife, we were finally in the labour ward at the Linkwood Clinic. We chose the Linkwood because the conditions there were the closest we could get to being at home. Partners could stay over, and the room had an en suite bathroom with a bath large enough for me to have the water birth we wanted.

Oliver was a week late in coming, so I was induced at midnight. Four hours went by: no pain, no discomfort, no labour. Four hours later Phindi suggested that we rupture the amniotic membrane. My waters broke, but still there was no pain and no labour. After yet another four hours, Phindi thought it best to add some intravenous induction medication. Still nothing happened. Oliver's heartbeat was persistently strong and regular. But it had now been nearly sixteen hours, with four-hourly medical intervention, and still he hadn't come.

Very gently Phindi, whom by now we were calling Ms Another Four Hours, suggested that we consider an epidural. While the prospect of no pain was appealing, we were disappointed that I wouldn't be able to give birth in water. Albie, constantly supportive, had been ready to change into his swim-shorts to help receive the baby! But we both accepted the new approach. We didn't want to jeopardise Oliver's chances of a safe and uncomplicated arrival.

The anaesthetist was called to administer the epidural. Halfway through the procedure, all of Joburg suffered a power blackout and he had to complete the task by the light of his cellphone! A few hours later, still no Oliver.

When Phindi came back to monitor my progress, she said the inevitable: 'I think you'd better have a Caesar.' It was crushing to hear it, but we knew it was for the best. The waiting was almost over. But now there was another obstacle. We were ready, but the building wasn't. The power was still off. The operating theatre was on the ground floor and we were up on the second. The elevators were not working, but the theatre was in full swing with another C-section under way. My turn was next. The paramedics were called to help carry my bed down the big winding staircase. Suddenly, in a scene reminiscent of *MASH*, orderlies came rushing into my room, unplugged the drips, secured the sides of the bed so I wouldn't roll off, and, with a drip on wheels careering at my side, we went flying down the corridor. By then the elevator was working again, so they decided to go the quicker route. But what if the lift got stuck with me in it? Fortunately the power held out, and five seconds later the doors opened to an anxious-looking Albie, who had taken the stairs.

In the theatre we were surrounded by Dr Somaya Ebrahim and her assistant; Dr Marianne Lucic, the paediatrician; Dr Patrick Wong, the anaesthetist; Phindi Mashini, who didn't need to stay, but wanted to be there for the birth; and Ben Viljoen, our photographer friend. Together we were a fair representation of the United Nations. A guessing game started about how big Oliver might be. As Somaya made the incision, someone made a joke about the risk of a skew cut line with legal eyes watching and a photographer present to capture the evidence. We laughed. Somaya made a poignant comment about the joy of cutting to bring life and not to remove disease. It all added to the drama of the moment. Then suddenly Somaya exclaimed, 'My gosh, what a big head! What a big baby!' A dignified little yowl, a quick wipe and then he was on my chest. Albie and I both cried. And no one had guessed anywhere near 4.64 kilograms!

○

Postscript
Driving to work along Oxford Road soon after Oliver's birth, I was startled and amused to see posters announcing 'Sachs word pa op 71'.[1] It suddenly hit home that at this late stage in my life I had become a father for the third time. Never had I wished for something so definitely, so intensely. And yet I felt suddenly anxious that I wouldn't measure up. Being a father to my older sons, Alan and Michael, had given me great joy. But they were now in their mid-thirties. It was a long time since I'd experienced the demands of being father to an infant. I believe in shared child-rearing. Yet my work as a judge requires long, concentrated hours into the night. Would I be able to help Vanessa enough?

---

1 'Sachs becomes a father at 71'.

These were my rational concerns. But there are moments when your heart speaks louder than reason: the positive result with the home pregnancy kit; the little wriggling bits on the scan; the skill, compassion and cultural diversity of the medical team attending Oliver's delivery; the feeling that we were witnessing, alongside his birth, the birth of a new country – not only a more just but a more generous and expressive one; finally, that great moment – his affirmative first cry as he emerged and was placed on Vanessa's breast. I felt elated and ready for anything.

Soon after Oliver's birth, a journalist asked sympathetically, 'Can we say you are a proud father?' I found myself objecting to the word 'proud'; it seemed just too patriarchal. Proud of my seed? Proud of producing an heir? I was a joyous parent with a huge bonus in life, not a proud producer.

The sleepless nights I had feared did not happen. I'm usually a light sleeper, but the three of us slept soundly in bed together. Oliver was so quiet. In those first weeks I would get closer to make sure he was still breathing. He would wake and suckle and sleep again.

Now that he is older, the intense companionship and shared fun and delight give me added energy for my work. My anxiety over the superfluity of happiness has not completely vanished, but the joy continues. There is something of this feeling in an American lullaby I sing to our son at night:

I gave my love a cherry that has no stone,
I gave my love a chicken that has no bone,
I told my love a story that has no end,
I gave my love a baby with no crying.

How can there be a cherry that has no stone?
How can there be a chicken that has no bone?
How can there be a story that has no end?
How can there be a baby with no crying?

A cherry when it's blooming it has no stone,
A chicken when it's pipping it has no bone,
A story of I love you it has no end,
A baby when it's sleeping has no crying.

Stone-Washed Buildings

Imraan Coovadia

Yale–New Haven Hospital at 20 York Street in New Haven, Connecticut, has the distinction of being the birthplace of President George W. Bush. George W. was born to George and Barbara Bush on 6 July 1946. After the 2000 presidential election, the town installed a signboard advertising this fact on the long highway which follows the shoreline past New Haven all the way up to Canada in one direction, and all the way down to Florida in the other. Last I heard, the board had been taken down. You can't rely on America's goodwill. On a smaller scale, you certainly can't rely on New Haven's favour. Its most famous mayor, Benedict Arnold, was the most notorious traitor in American history. Many of the buildings at Yale were constructed during the Great Depression by out-of-work Italian artisans. They first buried the stones for a year in an underground limestone pit so that the dormitories and colleges would have a suitably weathered appearance. Later, people would do the same thing with denim. In the United States, which has been postmodern since 1776, history is a matter of appearances. If a date has to be fudged or a building has to be weathered, so be it.

Yale–New Haven isn't only the birthplace of George W. Bush. My son Zaheer was born there – as it happened, during the election recount on 18 November 2000. I call him Zaheer, but in fact his name was just as closely contested as the vote totals were in Florida, and he was to remain nameless for some time after his birth. His mother's family, who were immigrants to the United States from St. Petersburg, had determined that he should be Russian, and Jewish, and as fanatically conservative as they were. I didn't agree. They had rebelled against their own parents who had been members of the KGB, but they hadn't rebelled against the peremptory KGB style. So it was logical

49

that I began to think of them as a sort of secret police who had gained access to my existence. But perhaps this is not all that unusual with in-laws.

Coincidences, like sorrows, come in threes. The paediatrician we saw at Yale–New Haven had trained with my father at King Edward Hospital in Durban. (We can call this woman Cecily because I cannot for the life of me recall her actual name.) Cecily, or Gwendolyn if you prefer, had no trace of a South African accent. She had been a medical student at what was then the University of Natal and admired my father from a technician's point of view. She remembered that he had been able to inject two dozen children around the ward in the time it took an American physician to do one child. (It's often this way, I think. Although the Third World is supposed to be riddled with inefficiency, stupidity and corruption, and it may well be, it's frequently the case that a country like South Africa can't afford the scale of inefficiency and incompetence that a wealthy nation can.)

Apart from her point about the injections, there was no other line of conversation that Cecily, or Gwendolyn, proposed. She was a lackadaisical doctor as well as a lackadaisical talker. We happened both to have grown up in Durban, but it might as well have been in different sections of the galaxy. In the cosmic sense, maybe we were simply passing through Durban at the time of our respective births. I guessed it would have taken Cecily and her family about sixty years to move in stages from Vilnius in Lithuania to New Haven or the town of Orange in Connecticut.

South Africans living overseas tend to vanish into the environment, into one or another generic category. This meant that, unlike my in-laws, I had no idea what sort of identity I should transmit to my son. Having a child raises the issue of tradition in its purest form, and it was clear that I had no answer to the paradoxes thus created. Even in more ordinary circumstances tradition is a moving target, new wine in old bottles. You read the labels on the bottles and pretend to be satisfied when, in fact, you can't raise a child, however you might wish to, in the vintage of your own childhood.

Names are an obvious part of this problem. All of our names were strange. I was named, I have it on good authority, after the Pakistani cricketer, although I can't bowl a cricket ball without dislocating my shoulder, and although I once served as the scorer for the First XI of my boarding-school cricket team without knowing if there were six or eight balls in an over.

Luba, Zaheer's mother, whose name is Russian for 'love', lived up to her own name as well as I lived up to mine. I wasn't at all sure if Luba cared for me. On balance, I thought not. She had decided that I was a dreadful writer. I thought I might like her, although it may have been that I was impressed by her looks and maybe more so by her runner's temperament. I could never get anywhere on my own two feet, having inherited the Indian disease of indolence and pyjama-wearing. Even while she was pregnant, fantastically pregnant, Luba ran half-marathons on the weekends. It took me about the same amount of time to shuffle the mile down Orange Street to the Yale campus.

Of course runners are dour, persistent, utterly inflexible human beings, but this fact about Luba (whose name in English can also be spelled 'Lyuba' and even 'Lyubov' when it is fully extended) impressed me. She had a mind as firmly entrenched in its opinions as the Red Army at Stalingrad, whereas my own thoughts and conclusions about the world were essentially naval in character: mobile, subject to external conditions and non-territorial. An army can't fight a navy and vice versa. They can only exchange barrages.

In fact this analogy between Luba and the Red Army has, as I have suggested, a solid basis in fact. Her grandfather was a Communist academician, which I regarded as a favourable indication. As a South African who in the early 1980s had read banned volumes of Engels and Lenin in the form of *samizdat*, I had a remaining romantic feeling about the Soviet Union. When I thought of Luba's family as the KGB I meant it in as fond a way as can be imagined.

The Russian Communists, as Milan Kundera likes to point out, were masters at erasing and revising the historical past.

Luba's KGB were every bit as energetic at their own forms of erasure. In this instance they were erasing me. The KGB organised a *bris*, a Jewish circumcision ceremony, and for a sum of five hundred dollars hired a *moyle*, an expert at circumcision who inserted a drop of kosher wine into the victim's mouth and then, exploiting his confusion, removed his foreskin with a device that resembled a cigar clipper. I was absorbed by the fact that this *moyle* was a woman. It was a dubious profession for a lady, too visible an articulation of hostility towards men.

Most of my life, I think, has involved leaving physical facts behind. (When Socrates defines philosophy as learning how to die, this is really what he means.) Women who experience pregnancy and birth don't have the same indulgence. The physicality of my son's birth astonished me. I made it to the delivery with ten minutes to spare. I had a headache from four hours of sleep under the influence of Stilnox. And yet, as Zaheer was handed to me like a book at a school prize-giving, I had the sense that I had never been so present at the scene of life. I'll never forget people's expressions, especially Luba's, but what they meant I still don't know if I can say.

Even though I did get there in time, I was certain, when I went to have the required bracelet placed on my son's wrist, that I had already failed in every other way as a father of one minute's standing. The first mental note I made was that the scope of my past and potential failures – failures to connect, to understand, to forgive, to acquire wisdom, to create something on a solid basis – had now spread from one life to two.

My father, whose wisdom is immense, had reminded me to register my son's birth with the South African embassy in case he needed a South African passport. I had other worries at the time, like writing a dissertation, and forgot. But my nameless and renamed son is sitting on the opposite side of the bed as I write this piece, and it strikes me that the birth of every child is the chance for a parent to be born again without the interposition of holy water.

When a Name is Lost

Epiphanie Mukasano

I remember the spasms in my left eye. They say in Rwanda that spasms on the lower lid mean crying and those on the upper lid mean receiving a gift. Which eyelid was it? I cannot tell now.

What I do remember is that it was a sunny Tuesday in July, in the long, dry season before the *umuhindo*[1] brought the rain and cooled the air. I was helping Adrian, our cook, with preparations for making sweet banana wine. We had a small banana plantation on our plot of land across the street from our house in Kimisagara, a suburb of Kigali. The bananas were ready to be cut down and buried in a pit to ferment. We had lined the pit with green banana leaves and were laying the bananas inside and covering them with soil. After five days, when they had fermented, we would go to the rain forests in the mountains to cut *ishinge*, a special grass through which we would press the banana juice. We would press and press until the sweet juice ran out. It made powerful wine, much stronger than the wine I have tasted here. Three bottles could get a big man rolling drunk. Making banana wine was important for us. It brought people together and kept them together.

I had just stripped some bananas from a branch, when I felt the first pangs. I was no novice. I had already given birth to two children and I knew I had to find a lift to the hospital soon. I couldn't go by taxi or bus; I needed the safety and reliability of a private car.

I left Adrian to fill the banana pit and walked to find my friend Judith, who lived in my neighbourhood. We were both teachers, enjoying our long school holiday. It had started at the end of June and would last until September. Judith reassured me

---

1 The *umuhindo* are the electric storms of early October.

that her car would be available whenever I needed to go.

I had already prepared the baby's suitcase. It wasn't big. In my country they say that you should not spend a fortune on an unborn baby. If you do, it could bring you bad luck. At around five in the afternoon my husband came back from town with building supplies. Like many people do before the birth of a child, we had been renovating our house. Seeing me doubled over, he ran to fetch Judith, and within minutes she was driving us to Centre Hospitalier de Kigali, one of the biggest hospitals in town.

It was only twenty minutes away, but the journey felt long. As I looked out of the car window, life on the streets was going on as usual. People were buying fruit and vegetables in the covered markets that you find all over Kigali, between the apartment blocks and houses.

My contractions were getting stronger. I shifted on the seat, trying my best not to make a noise, trying to prove myself a strong woman. We drove up the hospital driveway in the dry, dry heat, past the eucalyptus trees and the bright red bougainvillaea creepers to the hospital entrance. My husband and I had been together in the car, but when we reached the building, I had to go inside alone. It was hospital regulations. My husband could only visit; the hospital staff would phone him if there was an emergency. We didn't question this. It was common in Rwanda for men not to be present at the birth of their children. I didn't like it. I wanted someone I loved and trusted to be near me.

Judith and my husband comforted me and told me that everything would be all right. I waved as they drove away. I would see them again when they visited the next day.

I was on my own.

A nurse took me to a small room, where she examined me. She told me that the labour was still in its early stages. I did not believe her. I was in so much pain. She suggested that I walk around the maternity ward to encourage the contractions. The ward was full and noisy. I passed women screaming and swearing. It made me feel more nervous. There were so many women, but I still felt alone.

At around seven in the evening I was checked again. The progress was slow. About an hour later they decided to do a scan. I was told that the umbilical cord was wrapped around the baby's neck and that there was a danger of it strangling the baby if I tried to have a natural birth. I would have to have a Caesarean delivery immediately, under general anaesthetic. (They didn't do epidural Caesareans in Rwanda at that time.) I did not like the idea. I had heard stories about Caesars. You had to spend at least eight days in hospital, sleeping on your back. You could not eat before you had let out the accumulated gases, or else your tummy would burst, people said.

I was hurried to the theatre. A doctor and a team of nurses surrounded me. I was very scared. My first two sons had come out naturally. What if I didn't make it? As they gave me the injection, they explained to me that I wouldn't feel any pain at all. I remember my heart beating very fast. In that hospital in Kigali, the nurses comforted me and prayed for me as I sank into a twilight sleep.

The next morning, as I slowly regained consciousness, I saw a nurse standing next to my bed.

'You have a baby girl,' she said, laying the sleeping baby next to me.

I was overjoyed. I had really wanted a girl. Now I had my gift.

In Rwanda we name children according to the circumstances in which they are born. Or after what we wish for at the time. Or to honour the feeling we have when we first see our baby. Sometimes, if a baby is born in a difficult situation, we name them to remind us of this. Every child is given their own surname, chosen by their parents. This is very confusing for people living in South Africa, whose surnames are passed down from parent to child.

My father, who worked as a clerk in Muramba parish in Gisenyi, named me Epiphanie Mukasano. In a bookcase in his house, he had a very big book. It had all the names of the saints and the stories of their lives. When he had to find a Christian name, he went to that book. I think this is where he found my name, in the *Book of Martyrs*.

I didn't have to look in that book to name my daughter. When I saw her little chubby face for the first time, I saw no similarity between her and myself. She looked just like her father. And so for her first name I just had to add an *e* to her father's name, Celestin, to make *Celestine*. Celestine's surname would be very special: *Kampire*, meaning 'one who brings luck'.

My husband was delighted to have a daughter. Before I became pregnant for the third time, he had suggested we be content with two boys. But I had wanted four children. Now, he said, we can stop. You have your girl, you will be happy now, he told me.

I went home after a week in hospital. I was pleased to be back in my house with my family, and my boys were happy to have a sister. My sister-in-law looked after me. She helped bathe and change the baby. I was very spoiled. I was lucky to have her with me. It took time to heal from the Caesar, and I was impatient to carry my baby on my back, the way my mother had carried me. She had used the traditional sheepskin, wrapped together with a piece of cloth, the strips of skin tied around her waist. In our so-called civilised world, we were losing this tradition. We just used a piece of cloth. I used the same cloth to carry all my children, my two sons and now my daughter. I kept it over the years. I kept it from Rwanda to Cape Town. How sad I was to lose it last year, when I gave a bag of clothes to a crèche. It must have got mixed up with them.

I would sit in our yard in Kigali with my new baby in the shade of the tall cassava trees we call *ibucucu*. I used to cook the huge leaves from these trees together with meaty bones to make a stew. It was good for breastfeeding, as it encouraged the production of breast milk. We also had three huge avocado trees. Everyone had at least two or three of these in their yard. And sweet, small bananas called *kamara masende*, meaning 'money' (you buy and buy them until your pocket is empty). As she grew, I would feed my baby girl avocados with rice and those sweet bananas. I can still smell them. Although I have looked, I have never found them anywhere else.

We fled Rwanda in May 1994, when the war had got worse and our lives were in danger. When I heard that we had to leave,

I packed five suitcases. One contained all our precious family photographs wrapped up in our best clothes. Unfortunately, when the minibus came to fetch us, the driver told me that we couldn't take all the suitcases with us. Taking all five would mean leaving people behind. In that madness, I remember it being so difficult to decide what to leave behind, what to take. But the decision was made for me. The driver just grabbed the two nearest suitcases and threw them in the car.

We hoped that we would be back in a few months, at the most. We deserted our house, still full of furniture, the children's toys, the cot the baby had slept in, the kitchen cupboards with food uneaten, the television and radio, the buckets in the yard.

When I opened my two suitcases, I saw that they were full of old clothes. The one containing our family photographs had been left behind.

We moved from one place to another, hoping that the war would end soon. But when it became clear that it wasn't going to, we crossed the border. Celestine had her second birthday in the DRC.

◯

I watch my son and daughter as they walk between the shacks down the narrow, sandy track to the tar road. It is a long journey to school. A cold wind is blowing sand and litter everywhere. Dogs are looking for scraps in the rubbish bins on the street.

Celestine turns and waves. Soon she will be sixteen. She has grown up not knowing her country, not knowing her own name.

I go inside, out of the wind, and find an exercise book with her name on it. I open it and start to write down my memories of her birth, memories of our life then. I want to give this story to her for her sixteenth birthday. It is not easy to remember all the details, so many years later. The years of hardship seem to have eroded everything. But I must try, for her sake.

Celestine, I want to be able to tell you the story of where and how you were born. And where you got your special name. The name you find so difficult to pronounce. Celestine Kampire, you are the one who brings luck. The Rwandan meaning is very special – don't forget it.

A Knitted Cap

Maire Fisher

I want to get an early night – I have to be up with the sparrows tomorrow. I'm booked in for a Caesar, ten days short of my due date. I have no hang-ups about not giving birth naturally. After four miscarriages and one emergency Caesar, all I care about is that this new baby will arrive safely. I'm not a good incubator, conceiving easily but losing my babies before the end of the first trimester.

As I lean over to kiss Rob good night, I feel an intense pain. It's not a contraction. It doesn't feel right, nor does it go away. After a quick phone call to the gynaecologist, we drive at speed to the hospital. When we get there, there's no delay. I'm given an epidural and go straight to theatre. Rob scrubs up and puts on a surgical gown. He stands close to me and watches and takes photographs as our second son is delivered. They let me hold him for a brief moment and then I'm wheeled away to the recovery room. Rob stays while they clean our baby and perform all the tests. His Apgar scores are a perfect ten, Rob tells me when he comes through to join me.

Paralysed from the waist down, I feel no pain. I hold out my arms. Cocooned in a pale blue blanket, my son is handed to me. His skin is dusky, and I think he will not be as fair as his older brother. His head moves blindly to milk and then he coughs – a little rasping sound – and immediately my arms are empty. The faint warmth of his body lingers. All is sudden action, doctors on the scene. My blood rushes. My heart pounds.

They can't tell us too much – tests are being run, X-rays taken. I am helped into a wheelchair and taken in to see him. Small glass domes line sides of the neonatal ICU. Tiny babies, wizened faces, tiny hands like tiny birds' claws. My son is large, too healthy to be here. Except for the tubes feeding into and out of him. I have to wash my hands before I can reach out a finger to stroke him. Unlike the other babies, he lies in an open incubator. Above him a monitor chirps. Glowing lines peak, dip, peak. Fluorescent lighting turns the green of a surgeon's gown a surreal hue. Another monitor screeches, a high-pitched urgent whine. The hum of machines merges with the hum of voices. Nobody speaks loudly. Hushed action, hushed speed. Everything shines – white, sterile. Stainless-steel surfaces, impossibly clean.

Strange, small details hold the world in place. A thin tube carries white milky stuff to my son's stomach. An elastic band attached to a pale green knitted cap keeps the breathing tube wedged in his rosebud mouth. The cap looks home-made and I wonder who knitted this scrap of headgear. The cap is my focus. That and the feeble grasp of my baby's perfect fingers around my thumb.

Rob stands talking to the doctors. His face pale, he hears words like *oxygen*, *lungs* and *machines*. I hear the clicking and the beeping but nothing penetrates. Later I hear them in my dreams. We aren't allowed to stay too long. Again I'm pushed past the glass domes. Stick-like arms wave at us as we pass.

Back in my room, Rob and I stare at each other. 'He'll be fine,' I say. 'He's in the best place possible,' Rob says. Small comments to break the silence. I lie trapped in my bed, Rob paces the room. He speaks to the nursing staff, but there's no news. Eventually he has to go home, tell everyone what has happened. He bends to hug me. I run my hands over his back and hold on to him. He kisses me goodbye, says he will get back as soon as he can.

I'm alone in my room. I could use the phone, speak to my parents. But I don't want to. I don't have any words. I suck on an ice cube, but my mouth stays dry. They tell me to sleep, that they will let me know when I can see him. 'You need your rest,' they say. I think of Rob, hope he's managing to get some sleep. The night passes in a blur of semi-wakefulness, and each time I ask about my baby I am told not to worry, that I will see him in the morning.

Early the next morning the paediatrician arrives. He uses

simple words to explain the condition rooted in my womb and bred during the long months of incubation. He tells us about respiratory distress syndrome and hyaline membrane disease. Our baby's lungs are failing, and he's battling to breathe.

But there's hope. Hyaline membrane disease is caused by a lack of surfactant, a soap-like substance that coats the lungs. A modified natural pig-lung extract, Survanta, will increase his chance of survival dramatically. It's expensive, he warns us, and he needs our permission to go ahead with it. 'Yes, yes,' we both say. 'Anything, everything you can do.' Rob listens intently, but my stubborn mind won't hear the words *survival* or *complication*. All I want is to get back to the ICU.

When the paediatrician leaves a nurse comes to remove my drip. I clutch Rob's hand, using his firm grip to help me walk as fast as I can. Our son still lies in the open incubator. Another tube snakes into him, fed into the hole punched between his tiny ribs and into his chest cavity. This new tube acts as a drain and keeps his lung inflated. I hear another medical term – *pneumothorax*. Air had leaked into the space between his chest wall and the outer tissues of his lungs. When one lung collapsed during the night, the paediatrician performed emergency surgery, standing right where I am standing now. He resuscitated our son three times during the night. I remember now his red-rimmed eyes, how exhausted he looked when he spoke to us.

We spend hours staring at our baby, tracing the lines on the monitors, listening to the *blip – blip – blip* that guards his breath, his blood. His eyes are open, indigo, overlaid with a deep brown. He looks so much like Daniel did at birth, but we see the differences – his eyebrows are sparser, the shape of his eyes different. Although they both measured exactly the same – fifty-three centimetres – his body seems longer, less solidly compact than his brother's. And he is so quiet. Apart from his cry at birth and that small telling cough, I haven't heard him make a sound.

Eventually, Rob has to leave, beginning the endless shuttle between home and hospital, keeping things going. I cling to him. I don't want him to go. He doesn't want to leave. He's desperate to see Daniel; I'm desperate to know that Daniel is all right. He promises to come back as soon as he can, and to bring Dan with him. I promise to stay near our baby. But I can't, not the whole time.

I'm determined to breast-feed, and if I want to do this I will have to express every day, make sure that my milk comes in. I'm taken into a small cubicle, shown how to attach the suction pump to my breast. I switch on the breast pump, listen to its rhythmic suck and release. There isn't much, but what there is is thick and yellow, filled with all the good things a baby needs. I hate having to pour it down the sink. Hate the fact that a tube in a vein feeds him, sip by tiny sip.

Late that afternoon Rob brings Daniel to visit. Somehow he has also managed to fit in a trip to the registry office, and our son now has a name, Kieran Peter. It is wonderful to whisper 'Kieran' as we approach him, to tell Daniel to say hello to his little brother.

And then we wait, all our energy concentrated on one small body, one small chest, rising and falling.

Three days later, a milestone: Survanta, the miracle drug, is doing its job and Kieran is moved from the high-care open incubator to an intensive-care closed one. His teddy bear, a gift from Daniel, moves in with him, perched at the foot of the incubator.

The haze of hospital days passes, one into another. Hospital time is different from outside time. Everything slows. Hospital time balloons, then shrinks to a moment of satin skin, stroked by one finger inserted through a plastic framed chink. I feel these seconds with every whorl of my fingertips. Suspended in hospital time, dangling on threads of hope and fear, we wait. For doctors to complete their rounds, for nurses to break from routine and give us the latest details. In this other world, only the waiting matters.

Each day the ICU staff tell us we should take photos of Kieran. But somehow, between us we manage to block out this instruction. I don't remind Rob to bring the camera; he forgets it yet again.

Friends and family visit. I speak to them, but cannot remember what I have said. The only times that feel real are the early evenings when Rob brings Daniel to see me. We walk out into the fresh air, the green gardens, and he tells me about his day. I play with him, read to him as he perches on my bed. When it's time for them to leave, I want to hold Daniel tight, not let him go home.

They tell me that I should rest more. But I don't want to rest, hate lying in that bed. I ask Rob to bring me some proper clothes. Showering each morning, then dressing, gives me something to do. I even put on make-up, stroke colour into my cheeks and onto my lips. I do this quickly, avoid looking into the mirror for too long, because I am not sure that the woman who stares back is me. Everyday tasks – washing, eating, dressing – are performed by the stranger who has taken over my body. The one who smiles, says 'Thank you', talks to the nursing staff, learns the names of the other parents who haunt the ICU. Perfectly under control, or so she thinks.

Until the day they tell me that someone will be joining me in my semi-private ward. I am there by default as it is. I'd been booked into a general ward, but this one had been free, and so they'd put me here, away from all the mothers who have their babies with them. I crack. I won't, I will not, I cannot share my room with a nursing mother. I don't rant or rave or scream. Instead I burst into tears and ask if they can move me to a private ward. By this stage the thought of what all this is costing has ceased to matter. It's become another of the things to be dealt with – after. They don't move me from my room, nor does anyone come to share it with me.

One day, the eighth I think it is, they tell me I have to leave but Kieran has to stay. I am not sick and a hospital is no place for a healthy person. I need to go home and visit Kieran, instead of staying in the insulated world of the hospital. I protest. 'I can't leave him,' I say. 'How can you ask me to leave him?' But they are firm; they tell me we will cope better this way. I walk slowly down the passage, feeling as though the air has been sucked from my lungs, my stomach filled with stones. Alone in my room, I cry for a long time. Then I get up from my bed and pack my bags.

It takes a day or two to settle but it feels right to be home, to become part of my family again. Rob and I split our days between son and son. We both sleep better. Life feels almost normal: cooking meals, bathing Dan, singing him to sleep. One day I find myself laughing – for the first time since Kieran was born.

I spend hours on the phone, giving family and numerous friends updates on Kieran, but can't fully explain what is wrong with him. I have no desire to explore the ins and outs, the implications of his illness. I have the gist of it, enough to give a potted idea of what his condition means. 'Think of his lungs as being like a perished rugby ball,' I say.

Each day, Kieran improves. His weight creeps up, but still I am not allowed to hold him. And each day, when I ask when I will be able to, I'm told – kindly, patiently – to wait. 'He's doing well,' they say. 'Soon, soon.' I want to take the clock hands and force them to move faster, but at the same time I know that each hour, each day Kieran spends here, he is becoming stronger.

I get to know the ICU staff better, have more time to watch them as they work. One of the sisters tucks a premature baby inside her uniform, against her skin. They need as much body contact as possible, she tells me. A corkboard near the nurses' station is covered in photographs – a collage of babies who have been cared for here. Babies held by their moms and dads. I imagine Kieran's photo up there – he is a perfectly beautiful baby – but we still do not bring the camera to the ward.

The last of the tubes is removed. The sister on duty opens the incubator and – for the first time in sixteen days – we hold our baby boy. Feather-light. Vulnerable. Exposed. I am petrified. What if he picks up one of the infections that are surely lurking, waiting to attack him? Kieran lies in my arms and I take a deep breath. Rob reaches forward to stroke his cheek. And then he shifts his chair closer and I hand him his son to hold. We don't say much – we murmur to Kieran, tell him how beautiful he is. And he murmurs back.

My milk, which I have been expressing faithfully every day, lets down and my shirt is soaked. The sister tells me that I can try to feed him tomorrow. Once he is feeding properly we can take him home. It shouldn't take more than a couple of days, she says. Rob and I leave in a daze, not quite sure that what we have heard can possibly be true.

I arrive at the hospital early the next morning. The sister places Kieran in my arms and I feel again a surge of panic, a drenching of fear-filled sweat. I lift my T-shirt, fumble with the hooks on my bra and guide my nipple to his mouth. He roots, snuffles and latches. A small splutter as his mouth fills and then he settles. One hand kneads my breast; the other grasps my thumb. Something shifts inside me, a feeling of things being as they should be. I move him to my other breast, and gradually his sucking slows, his hands still, his eyes close. I hold him while he sleeps. Then gently, gently, I place him back in the incubator. I flop back into the chair, wrung out. Then I leap up again and rush to the payphone. I call Rob, and when he answers I burst into tears. His voice is urgent, concerned. He tells me to slow down, tell him what the matter is. 'Sorry,' I say. 'Sorry. Nothing's the matter. I fed him, and nothing's the matter!'

For the next few days I stay at the hospital for as long as I can, feed Kieran as often as I can. On the twentieth day, Rob and I are both there when the paediatrician comes to beam his approval of how well Kieran is doing. He asks us to pop in to see him on our way out.

When we get to his rooms he tells us to pack a bag with baby clothes, because tomorrow Kieran will be going home.

○

Remembering is difficult. Until now I haven't written much about Kieran's birth. Some details remain hidden, buried thirteen years deep. Others, such as the discovery that not one of the photos Rob took in the operating theatre came out, still have the power to devastate.

But remembering brings joy, too. Rob and I have two precious sons. Our miracle babies. Miracles of technology, miracles of medical expertise. How can I fully express how I feel about them, explain all they bring to our lives? Is any parent ever able to find the words to describe those moments when love clenches your heart and stops your throat and all you can do is grab a passing son, hug him, then hug him harder and say, 'Oh, I do love you!'

The Tap

Troy Blacklaws

I'm in a pub called The Tap in Sherborne, Dorset. Two pints down. Pool balls clink like castanets. A feeling akin to vertigo spins my head. I stare at the speck in the V of the hazy scan photograph sent in the post from Frankfurt. I can't picture myself as a father. I beg my English philosopher friend, Finn, for wisdom.

– What do I do? Do I give up my teaching post and go to Germany? How will I survive there? And then there's the language with its hard grammar and gob-hawking *r*'s. And then there's *her*. I find her sexy. She was cool on the beach in Greece and on our travels through South Africa . . . but won't shifting in with her lock-stock kill the magic?

Finn orders another round of flat, foamless beer.

– At least the beer's good in Germany, I go on. And there's good bread. But the winters are long and bitter. And humour's scarce.

– I'll give it thought, he tells me. It's not a simple matter.

A week of unfocused teaching and staining papers with coffee and dropping the ball into the tennis net goes by. All this time I imagine Finn pondering the question.

We rendezvous in The Tap again.

– So Finn. Your verdict?

– On what?

– On the question of the baby?

– Huh?

– On my becoming a father.

Finn gags on beer.

– Hey, Troy, sorry. I forgot.

– You forgot?

– Maybe the beer went to my head.

I realise I'm alone in this. I phone her from a call box in the pub to tell her I'll come to Germany and be a father to this photographed smudge.

○

The fecund arc of her belly mimics the curve of the front of the lurid orange VW Beetle flying along the forbidden bus lane in Frankfurt. We go past scowling Germans in stoic cars standing in Indian file at the bidding of the red light. The thing I fear beyond being caught by the *Polizei* is the kitsch, filmic horror of him being born in the car. Fortunately he (I have seen him in a black-and-white doctor's movie jigging his bony hand at me) has not yet surfaced by the time we abandon the VW in front of the hospital.

They tell her that she still has a long way to go. They strip her and put her in a bath and force her to listen to new-age, ambient music and to stare into a lava lamp. In the end, things go too fast for the nurses. They can't pick up the baby's heartbeat. One of the spasms just won't ebb (or fade, or let go, or whatever it is spasms do) and it's killing him. They yank her to her feet and frogmarch her to another room. The sliding door shuts me out.

When it opens they have drawn a crude crayon line from her navel downwards. She's tied down and her knees are clamped akimbo. A doctor comes running in, wearing jeans. He's had no time to don white or green (or whatever colour German doctors wear in theatre). When the door slides ajar again (in what's becoming a macabre slide-show, or a scene shot by Kubrick) I see him standing over her with a scalpel in hand. I hear her shout (in German): *Don't cut yet! I'm still awake!*

The door shuts again. I stand outside: sidelined. I imagine the blade slicing through the convex canvas of her skin. Next time the door slides I see the sliced-watermelon neatness of the cut. The doctor, catching my eye, yells at the nurses to get rid of him (being me).

But the nurses have scalpels and tubes and swabs to juggle. They merely frown at me and slide the door to.

For a long time the door stays shut. I realise how deeply I love her.

Then a nurse comes out and tells me *the baby* survived. I interpret this as telling me that *the mother* is dead. I stand there in a daze until the nurse appears again. She's holding him. His wary blue eyes gaze out of a folded, old-man's face. He is covered in a film of blood. He's beautiful.

I am left alone with him in my hands. I see her in his eyes. He squinches his eyes and yowls. Instinctively, I sing to him Zulu fragments from my boyhood. I run out of Zulu and sing 'Blowin' in the Wind'. He goes calm. His eyes check me out, spooking me.

I carry him onto a balcony and hold him up to the cold, blind-eye sky, African style. Then I fold him in my rugby jersey and begin to sob for her, gone, and us two alone in this foreign, frowning world.

The nurse comes to scold me. It's too cold outside for him.

Inside, she lies corpse-white on a trolley. I see her fingers twitch against the white sheet. I realise she's not dead, after all.

After they send me home, I go to a bar. I order a beer. I want to tell the barman that I've just become a father, but then change my mind. I stare into the glowing, fizzing amber of the beer and feel the euphoria alone.

○

Ten years after. I'm playing *boules* with coins on a beach on Ko Lanta, Thailand. It's me and Finn (my son, named after the English Finn) and his sister. The dying sun paints our skin orange. I tell them:

– Watch and learn from your old man.

Then I toss a coin far from the target, a bit of driftwood acting as the jack. They both giggle cuttlefish teeth. There's no drug that gives you this kind of high. And I wonder what kind of fool I was to waver then, long ago, in a dingy pub in Dorset called The Tap.

Positive

Nolubabalo Gloria Ncanywa

When I was a little girl I wanted to be a nurse. I would rip the white pages out of my exercise books and fold them to make paper nurse's hats. (In the old days the nurses used to wear white dresses and caps. I loved their uniforms so much.) My hair was wild and long, just the right place for a nurse's hat to sit. My teacher would scold me for tearing out precious paper, but my mother would look at me and say, 'Gloria, one day you will be a nurse.' And when I looked in the mirror I would see Gloria the nurse.

I wanted to be a nurse, but I didn't want to have anything to do with blood. If you showed me a cut or a person bleeding, I would run away screaming.

In the village in the Eastern Cape where I grew up, the men used to leave home to go and work in the mines in Johannesburg. My dad was one of them. He would disappear on the bus with all the other men, and only come back at Easter and Christmas. We would run out to meet the bus when it stopped, all dusty from travelling so far. The men would get off and look around for their families. I knew that when my dad came back from the mines, there would be money for food.

Life in my village was simple when I was a child. I lived with my mom and my two sisters and two brothers. I was the oldest. I used to fight with my sisters, then make up. There was lots of crying and laughing. We didn't have toys, not like the ones you buy in shops. We used to go to the dam nearby and dig red clay and make cows and dolls and sit in the hot sun by the water.

When I was thirteen, my mom got TB. I took care of her every morning before I went to school. When I came home I would lie next to her in her bed for hours, hugging and comforting her. When the TB got worse, she had to go to hospital for six months. I became the adult in the house, the one who had to look after the children. But then I got TB too, and had to go to hospital.

In the hospital I saw what the nurses did. Now I didn't want to be a nurse just so that I could wear the nice white uniform and the white cap. I saw that nurses helped people. If I could be a nurse, I could help my mother.

When I was better, my teacher wanted me to go back to school. I was a bright girl, but I was still looking after my mom. My father wasn't supporting us at that time. So my younger sister took my school books to use, and I stayed at home, only going back to school the following year.

In our village people got sick and died. I never questioned why. (It was only much later, when I knew better, that I would remember Mrs So-and-so or Mr So-and-so, and think they must have died of AIDS.) In our village AIDS did not exist. It was witchcraft – something people cursed you with, not something you got from unprotected sex. And sex was something we young girls talked about, but didn't practise. I was innocent then.

Children in rural areas are different. We grow up quickly physically, but we stay innocent for longer. My girlfriends and I were still playing with dolls, but we had dream boyfriends who would become dream husbands. My dream husband didn't drink or smoke. He was a Christian. We had two children, and a big car. I pictured myself driving that car.

When I was fourteen I had my first boyfriend. I played netball, and there was a thing among us girls: we had to have a boyfriend who played rugby or soccer. My boyfriend played rugby and he was a boxer. I loved him so much; we were best friends. Sometimes we kissed, but that was all. I could talk to him about anything. We would sit together for hours and tell each other things and laugh a lot. We would go together to fetch water from the river or the dam. My mom used to be amazed when I came back with a fifty-litre water drum. 'You must be very strong,' she would say. I wouldn't tell her that he had carried it for me. He made me happy. When we were late for school, we were late together. I thought he would be the one I would marry one day.

But it didn't happen like that.

In 1990, when I was sixteen, I met my husband. A woman, whom my father knew, came to our village. That woman asked me to help carry her bags back to her village. Her husband was away on the mines with my father. I helped the woman to carry her bags to the fence, which divided our village from the next one. When I reached the fence I told the woman that I needed to get home. It was six o'clock, the time everyone had to be home and I needed to cook. 'But there is no one to help me,' she pleaded with me.

At that moment I looked up and saw a man in the distance, waiting. I called him to come and help her, but he didn't hear, or he wasn't listening. When she saw that I wasn't going to go with her, she told me that I was going to be her brother's wife. It had been arranged. She had come to fetch me to take me to her village. I was still so young I thought she was joking, and I turned to go home. She let me go and I sang as I walked back along the path to my village, thinking that was it. All I had to do was to say no.

The road down the hill to my village is steep. There is a river between the fence, where I left the woman with her parcels, and the first huts of the village. I had crossed the river and was nearing the huts, when I saw five or six men, from my village, coming down the road towards me. Suddenly, I knew what was happening. But I still treated it lightly and was cheeky to them when I greeted them. They made a circle around me. They told me that they had been sent to take me to the next village to meet my husband. I refused to go. So they dragged me, crying loudly, back along the road.

When we got to the river they stopped. 'Let's leave her,' they said. 'She will get tired of crying and fighting soon.' They went and sat on the big rocks by the water. It was getting dark. I sat on the side of the road in tears, and waited. I was wondering why my family had not come out to look for me. The only reason the people in the village would not come out to help someone when they heard them crying was if they knew it was an arranged marriage. Then they would leave the girls to be taken to their husbands, because it was 'in our culture'.

I sat for a long time before the men came back and led me to the next village.

No one was going to rescue me.

When I saw my arranged husband, I didn't like what I saw. He was very fat. He was also twenty-four. I had seen him in church. Anyone that old, in church, was like a father to me. I was so young. I was still enjoying being a teenager with my girlfriends.

On that day, 26 October 1990, I was changed out of my old clothes, into the blanket the *makoti*[1] wore. With that change of clothes, at the age of sixteen, I married my husband and everything changed. Even my name. Nolubabalo became Nomilile. I hated the name, I hated the marriage and I hated being separated from my family, my friends and my boyfriend. I missed talking to him so much.

My husband went to Joburg and I stayed in his village with his family. I cried a lot. Before he went, he didn't force me to have sex, although his family were shouting at him to consummate the marriage. There was a belief that if a man had sex with his wife, she wouldn't run away. I didn't run away, but I refused to leave school. I told him before he left that if he didn't allow me to continue at school, I would leave him.

He came back in December. I had gone with his sisters to fetch water at the river. I remember looking up as they cried out, 'Milly, our husbands are home.' I saw three men coming towards us down the road. For the first time I thought, oh my goodness, he is my husband, I will have to have sex with him.

I was the only wife in the yard; we were alone in the house, as his sisters had moved to their houses. This is when the trouble started. On that day he came home, he asked me to bring water to wash. I took him the water, as that is what wives do. It was the middle of the afternoon. When I handed him the water, he closed the door. He wanted to consummate the marriage. I let him have sex with me. It wasn't nice at all. His sisters had said

---

1 'Married women'.

it would be nice. It was not. When I told them later, they said it was just because it was the first time. They told me that if I did it every day, it would be fine. It was not fine.

I confronted him. 'If you make me have sex, I will go home,' I said. He laughed at me. 'Your mother knows we are having sex,' he said. 'Your parents arranged this. But I won't force you.' That night he kept his word. But his word lasted only two days.

In 1992 he got a job in Port Elizabeth, and I spent my time between there and my home. I was still at school. The sex began to get better – he didn't force me any more – but I didn't get pregnant. Everyone waited for a baby. What was wrong with him? What was wrong with me? I told him that I didn't want a baby and he accused me of using contraception.

In 1993 I fell pregnant. But I had a miscarriage. I was nineteen and doing grade 11. The following year, when I was doing my matric, I fell pregnant again. This time I had to drop out of school. On 21 October I gave birth to my first-born, a boy. A beautiful baby boy. I gave birth in a hospital in P.E. The labour was very difficult. It started on a Sunday. My waters broke the following Thursday and I gave birth the next day. The first time I had sex I had pain, but this was like nothing compared to my labour pains. I had never felt such pain. When my husband saw how much I suffered, he said, 'This is the first and last baby.' He was kind to me. I had grown to love him over the years. I had forgotten about my dream husband with the big car; I had forgotten about my boyfriend I had sat and talked to for hours.

My husband didn't force himself on me any more and I had fallen in love with him. I was growing up. One day, he saw this. He looked at me and said, 'You see, you love me now, I can see it in your eyes.' I denied it.

When our baby was five months old, my husband started to cheat on me. I was so sad. It hurt so badly. He couldn't hide it from me. I knew when he had a new girlfriend. In December I went home to show my parents our little boy. They loved him. I was happy there in my village surrounded by my family. But

I went back to P.E. I wanted to talk to my husband, to tell him I was unhappy. But I couldn't, so I wrote him a letter, asking him questions – many, many questions. *Why are you doing this to me?* I asked. He read the letter and said he was sorry. But his being sorry didn't stop him for long.

In 1996 I went back to school and passed my matric. My boy was two. He made me laugh. He brought me joy. I didn't enjoy my marriage, but I enjoyed being a mother to my son. In 2000 my husband moved to Cape Town for work. I came to join him in the June holiday and got a job in a restaurant. But I told him I was going to return home after the holiday. I told him we couldn't live together. I knew that it would be all right for a few months, then we would start to fight, and so I was going to return home to my family in the Eastern Cape with my son.

On the morning I was due to leave, we went to church in Khayelitsha, where I was staying with my husband. I had packed my suitcase and a box of *padkos*[2] for the journey. When we got back from church, my husband started to eat my *padkos*. I told him it was for my journey, but he said he was hungry. Then he looked at me and asked me, 'Please stay with me. I don't want you to go.'

'We will fight,' I told him.

'I'm begging you,' he said.

And so I stayed. He was my husband, the father of my child.

I found a job as a security guard, and that June I fell pregnant again. This time I went for antenatal care. They asked me at the clinic if I would volunteer to have an HIV test. They said they were offering this service to all expectant mothers. I agreed. There was nothing to worry about. I hadn't been with other men. I was confident.

I remember the day I went back for the result. It was a sunny day. The sky was blue. But the result changed everything. It was positive. Everything just turned dark. I felt there was no hope at all. I was so scared I wanted to kill myself. As I made the journey

---

2 'Food for the road'.

home to Khayelitsha to tell my husband, I asked myself: What have I done to God? Why is he punishing me? Am I going to give birth to a dying baby? What are people going to say?

My husband was very supportive and concerned about our unborn baby. He didn't want it to suffer. We talked for a long time. What were we going to do with a sick baby? I was going to die. I would have to leave one orphan, my son, but did I want to leave two? We decided to terminate the pregnancy.

When I went back to the clinic, they told me it was too late. I was six months already.

At thirty-four weeks, I was given AZT to take twice a day. Then, when I went into labour, I had to take it three-hourly. In the hospital they checked my blood pressure. It was very high. I remember the doctor asking me what I was thinking, telling me to try to relax. They were kind to me in the hospital. I gave birth to a big baby boy. When I looked at him, I remember the nurses asking me, 'What do you wish him to be?' I didn't answer. He was going to die, I thought. What did it matter what I wished for him?

I remember looking at him and thinking he looked exactly like his father. When my husband came into the ward, he took our baby boy in his arms and said, 'He is so beautiful. He looks so healthy.' I looked at the other babies in the ward, then at my son. He was bigger. Surely this meant he was well? I comforted myself and convinced myself that he would live. I had to wait nine months to be able to test him for HIV. The test itself took only twenty minutes. The result: negative. He would live.

I remember coming home with him. There were people in the house. I went to my bedroom and prayed. When I came out, they asked me what had happened. I said, 'I am so happy, that's all I will say. Just keep it like that.'

Since then my life has changed so much. With my next pregnancy, I joined mothers2mothers, a support group for HIV-positive women. I knew, from my second child, that mothers can help protect their babies from the virus by taking the right medicine during pregnancy and labour, and by feeding correctly, not mixing breast and formula milk. I had protected my baby boy this way. I was stressed because of my status, and because I had not checked my CD4 count for three years, but I knew that I could protect this baby too. I also knew that the women at mothers2mothers would not judge me for falling pregnant. This, and knowing that I could get the treatment for the baby, made me strong.

I remember my excitement when I found out that it was a baby girl. I did my CD4 cell count. I couldn't believe it when it was 1579. A normal CD4 count is about 600–1500 cells. That's when I started to relax.

My baby girl was beautiful. I couldn't wait nine months to test her, as I had done with my son. I couldn't even wait six weeks. I tested her when she was four weeks. She was also negative. She cries like a bird, but I can't complain. I am enjoying being a mother to a baby girl.

In 2002, mothers2mothers started a group at the clinic in Site B, Khayelitsha. I was selected as a mentor mother, to give strength and support to other HIV-positive women. Soon I became a site coordinator for a team of mentor mothers. I worked every day at the clinic. This year I have been promoted to the head office in Cape Town, where I am a support administrator for the regional manager of the Western Cape.

My mother still lives in her village in the Eastern Cape. But things have changed there too. There are clinics where people are learning about HIV/AIDS. My mother is proud of me, of my family and my work.

When I look in the mirror now, I still see Gloria the nurse. I know it will happen, and I am planning to study again soon. Being HIV-positive has made me see things in a different way. I am no longer asking God why. I can see why.

Droëland

Ruth Ehrhardt

In memory of my mother

My mother, Carol Kathleen Ehrhardt, was born in Athlone in December 1950. In 1958, under the apartheid government's Population Registration Act, her family were reclassified from 'coloured' to 'white' and moved to a white residential area. My grandfather was a brilliant businessman, and in his 'new life' he quickly became a millionaire, enabling him to drive a Rolls Royce, travel the world first class and send his children to the best white schools.

My mother always resented this way of life. When she was eighteen, she saw her parents' offer to send her to finishing school in Switzerland as a way of escaping her identity as a 'white' South African. She lived in Switzerland for twenty years, studying for a doctorate in psychology and working as a social worker.

In 1979, the year before my birth, she chose to be reclassified 'coloured'. My younger sister and I grew up with her songs and stories of home, surrounded by the snowy mountains of Switzerland.

We moved back to South Africa in 1988 and my mother went in search of her lost 'coloured' family. She met my stepfather, who was trading in scrap metal and picking buchu in the mountains for a living. Together they bought the farm Droëland,[1] outside Ceres, and had two daughters. Their dream was to have a piece of land that would be both a sanctuary and a place of emancipation for the coloured people of South Africa.

My mother began to work with the farm workers, an oppressed and largely illiterate community. She became a counsellor to

---

1 'Dry land'.

them and a dispenser of medicine. She held church services with them, buried them and delivered their babies by candlelight.

'Droëland' is the story of the first baby my mother ever delivered on the farm. After that, pregnant women in the community chose not to go to hospital to give birth; instead they sent for her, trusting her able hands and soothing words. She delivered more than twenty babies on the farm.

When I became pregnant in 2001, my mother was my chosen midwife. She is the first person to have touched my eldest son.

On 26 May 2007, my mother, my stepfather and my seventeen-year-old sister, Gypsy, were killed in an accident on Michell's Pass, outside Ceres. It is to my mother that I dedicate this story, because I miss her so.

○

It is the middle of winter and the middle of the night. The wind moans and rain rips through the sky, stinging the windscreen, making it impossible to see.

My mother drives slowly along the farm road. The bakkie bumps and rattles over the rocks. Streams have turned to torrents of water, nearly impassable, and mud splatters the windscreen. She is driving down to one of the workers' cottages, where Hester is in labour.

She has her little enamel saucepan with her and the knitting cotton she bought back in Switzerland in the eighties. She also has black bags, towels, baby clothes, needle and thread, and a pair of scissors.

Hester is Willem Prins's wife. She is twenty-three, small and pretty, with high-cheekboned Bushman features. She had arrived a week earlier from Sutherland, heavily pregnant and travelling on a *donkiekar*[2] with her husband.

My mother drives into Ou Vloer,[3] the bottom part of Droëland, the part which dips into the Klein Karoo. She

---

2 'Donkey cart'.
3 'Old floor'.

continues through the gateposts and past the dam, full now from the rains.

She stops next to the little clay house with its lone pomegranate bush, grabs her bag of goods and the saucepan, and dashes through the rain. Willem Prins opens the cottage door, looking nervous.

'*Naand, mevrou.*'[4] He lets her in.

Inside the little house it is snug and warm and clean. The place is swept, the renosterbos broom leans in a corner against the wall. There is a foam mattress on the floor, and a small selection of baby clothes, white and neatly folded, lie on a makeshift shelf next to a pile of dark adult ones.

My mother draws aside a threadbare curtain hanging in a doorway and enters the bedroom. Hester is there on her knees, moaning softly to herself. A candle flickers in a coffee tin. The smell of protea logs burning in the fireplace fills the room. The firelight reflects in the beads of sweat on the young woman's brow.

My mother stands and quietly watches Hester as she kneels on the blanket. This is the first time my mother has experienced somebody in labour like this. She has read about it, but she herself has only ever given birth lying on her back with a monitor strapped to her.

Hester is frightened. She realises that her labour is not going well, that something is not right. My mother offers to drive her into town to the hospital, but Hester refuses. She has an outstanding account there, and she knows that they will refuse her entry unless that bill is settled.

Willem walks in and out of the room restlessly, but says and does nothing. He can hardly look at his wife. My mother decides to give him something to do. She hands him her enamel saucepan and asks him to boil some water.

The storm continues to batter the small, boarded-up windows.

My mother sits with Hester, rubbing her back as she writhes

---

4 'Good evening, Madam.'

about on the floor on all fours. My mother is whispering soothingly to her when there is a loud knock on the door. Ewert, a farm worker who has walked for kilometres in the rain, comes in wet and wild-eyed. He says that he is here to help, to teach my mother what to do. He tells her that he has delivered every one of his four children and cut their umbilical cords.

Ewert hands Hester a beer bottle and tells her to blow into it. This helps, and her feeling of hopelessness abates. Her focus is on her slow, rhythmic breathing, and no longer on the excruciating pain down there.

My mother whispers to Ewert that she feels something is wrong. Ewert agrees. He says that the baby is lying breech and that my mother must turn it around.

With the next contraction, my mother puts her large hand deep inside the pretty, delicate woman who is squatting and screaming.

My mother feels the slimy warmth of the woman's womb. Up she pushes, behind the child's back. Up, until she feels its soft little head. She turns the child. She turns it quickly before the umbilical cord wraps itself around its fragile neck.

The contractions become more intense and more frequent. Soon after, the head and the neck of the baby emerge.

Hester, still blowing into her lifeline, the brown beer bottle, clings to Ewert, sweating and moaning. And, with the next contraction, the rest of the baby's body slips out in a gush of mucus, water and blood.

A boy. A breathing baby boy.

After spluttering and coughing, he emits a soft, crackly wail. My mother wraps him in a towel and hands him to his bewildered mother, gesturing that she should now offer her breast to her son. The baby suckles eagerly. The young mother winces at the pain of the strong little jaws working away at her nipple.

The suckling brings on another contraction and with it the placenta is expelled.

Hester tore when my mother was turning the baby. Now my mother stitches her up. She advises Hester to visit the hospital as soon as possible, but she knows that she will never go.

Willem Prins, Hester and their little boy stayed on at Ou Vloer, on Droëland, for several months, working the flowers. But this work is seasonal, and when the winter months approached they moved on. So did Ewert, with his family.

Hester is dead now. Beaten to death by her husband.

Ewert wanders the streets with the *bergies*.[5] Still wild-eyed.

Whenever Hester's little boy sees my mother in the streets of Ceres, he runs up to her shouting excitedly, '*Ouma! Ouma!*'[6]

---

5   'Homeless people'.
6   'Granny! Granny!'

Mo

Rosamund Haden

At thirty-nine weeks pregnant I dance in slow motion across the grass. A friend, struggling to work my digital camera, captures a hibiscus flower, the wooden leg of a chair, an infinite expanse of summer sky and my billowing maternity dress.

Tomorrow I will go to hospital to have my baby boy. Feeling this imminent and terrifying responsibility, the child in me takes over, and I ham it up for the camera. Suddenly I am four again, the jester monkey copying my sister, exaggerating her moves as she dances seriously and beautifully to the record player in the garden of our family home.

That night, in the dark heat, I lie in bed with my hands on my pregnant tummy. The friends have gone, after wishing us luck. The camera is back on the shelf. But I can't sleep. We have just moved into a house near the sea and the rooms still feel unfamiliar. We have unpacked our boxes, hung up makeshift curtains and painted the walls. But, as a home, it doesn't feel permanent, not yet. It's as if we are on a seaside holiday. Perhaps it is the salt I can taste in the air, or the sandy garden where the plants grow close to the earth to counter the southeast wind.

At the foot of the bed, in the shadows, is our new pram. Next to it, on a chair, are the tiny jumpsuits that Thozama calls *rumbustas*, ready and waiting. It is close to midnight. I am aware that this might be my last night of proper rest for a long, long time, but for some reason this makes me less able to fall asleep.

It is strange knowing the day and approximate time that my son will be born. I try to imagine the new territory on the other side. A place where the comforting prospect of sleep will be replaced, I'm told, by a feeling of dread as night approaches. And where night itself will become indistinguishable from day. A place from which I should really turn and flee.

'What is it?' my husband asks, sensing my increasing anxiety.

I can't answer him.

'It's completely normal to be anxious before an operation. Everything will be fine. Just get some sleep.' He tries using his most reassuring voice, but I find it unconvincing.

'It's not about the Caesar,' I say, my voice high with tension.

'Take it easy.'

'I'm not worried about the operation. I'm worried about the baby. I'm worried that we haven't let him choose the time of his birth.'

I have had this anxiety ever since the doctor gave me two options for the Caesar date, 13 or 16 December. My husband has reassured me countless times that our son will not be scarred for life by our choice. He will be happy just to be alive and healthy. But as the date approaches my doubt resurfaces.

Every time someone asks when I'm due and I tell them I am having an elective Caesar, it feels like a confession. I add in mock alarm, '*Horror of horrors!*' in an attempt to pre-empt their reaction. I envy my husband's ability to disregard the opinions of others, especially those whom I have started to call, almost affectionately, the 'natural birth nazis'.

I listen as they tell me that I really shouldn't be doing this. That Caesar babies lack the ambition and drive of natural-birth babies. Something to do with not having pushed their way down the birth canal and out into the world. How could I miss out on the experience of natural childbirth? Surely I will regret it.

I remain quiet. I have my reasons. Although medical, none of them are likely to stand up before a natural-birth tribunal.

'Perhaps he would have held out until Christmas,' I continue in the dark, 'or been a midnight's child. Born when the hands of the clock joined.' I realise that I am talking to myself. My husband has fallen asleep next to me.

I lie back and close my eyes, but it's no use. I get up and open the window to let in some fresh air. Trying to fight back the first waves of panic, I tell myself to relax: 'Still your neurotic mind . . . let the random thoughts flow in and out.' The mantra from a meditation tape repeats itself over and over and my mind begins to play with the words, turning them upside down and back to front. Then an insane rhyme finds its way into my jumbled thoughts. A limerick a friend taught me with glee, when we were girls:

There was a young woman called Starkie
Who had an affair with a darkie
The result of her sins
Was quadruplets, not twins –
One black, one white and two khaki!

'Do you think he'll come out khaki?' I say in jest, hoping that by speaking I will regain some solid ground. But my husband has rolled over and is snoring. I don't persist. One of us should rest; one of us needs to be able to function in the morning.

I get back into bed, wondering what my grannies would say about me marrying a 'darkie' if they were still alive. For my British granny, Africans were the little black Sambos on marmalade jars. For my father's mother in Mpumalanga, they were strictly servants on her farm. They were *not* family.

I wonder what characteristics our son will inherit. What random genetic meetings will take place? Characters start to take shape on our family trees, illuminated in the dark. A lily-white, blue-blooded Sir Francis Dashwood peers down from the top branches, Chancellor of the Exchequer, founder of the Hell Fire Club. This nineteenth-century philanderer exits the folly at the bottom of the landscaped gardens of his stately home in High Wycombe, England, with its ha-ha and moon-shaped lake. High on opium, he staggers past a flock of sheep, back to his study for a nightcap before retiring. To procreate with reckless abandon?

Far away, around the same time in history, a pitch-black Xhosa tribesman of the Mfengu clan is forced to leave his settlement as the white timber merchants encroach into the heart of the Tsitsikamma forest. He leaves the canopy of massive yellowwoods for the Moravian mission station at Clarkson, near Port Elizabeth. The missionaries give him European clothes, a

Bible and the name *Swart Jong*.[1] His Xhosa name, along with his history, is lost down the generations. He marries Maria Goeda and our child's great-great-grandmother is born.

'There are so many la-di-f***ing-das in your family. Our son will be born with a silver teaspoon firmly lodged in his Settler mouth,' my husband likes to joke. 'As long as he doesn't grow up thinking everyone will pick things up after him.'

'Like his mother,' I add mechanically, before he can beat me to it. 'Don't forget my grandad was a humble parish priest. And your father is a Methodist preacher. You see, similarities!'

In the early hours of the morning, the ancestors are all around me in the room, dusting themselves off. Too many to accompany us in our car. Perhaps they have organised a taxi to the hospital to witness the birth. I picture them jostling for position over the bed, to get the first glimpse of an inherited likeness.

Will it be the determination and fiery strength of his grandmother, Maria Settler? Descended from Swart Jong and Maria Goeda, she had Malay, Indian and Mfengu blood mixed in her veins. By all accounts, she was a resilient, powerful person with a fierce sense of loyalty and a wicked sense of humour, inherited by my husband. Every now and then, needing a break from her life with her seven children, the clothing factory where she worked, and her own small business selling sweets and cooldrinks, she would escape by bus to a casino in the Ciskei, to do a bit of light gambling. On her tombstone is a simple inscription: *Sy doen wat sy kan*.[2]

Or will it be the adventurous nature of his great-great-aunt, Rosamund Everard King? Her obituary read: *First woman to fly a jet plane, wool queen, cattle judge, artist, aviatrix*.

I remember as a child finding a list written in her handwriting in an old farm ledger. It read: *cattle feed, fencing poles, if marry, make sure to take separate holidays, molasses* . . . I have often wondered whether if she had become pregnant before her husband died, she would have lived to be an old lady. On a

---

1 'Black Man'.
2 'She did what she could.'

sunny day one March she took her last solo flight. Her plane crashed, killing her instantly. It was a year after the war had ended.

Our son's great-grandfathers fought in the same war. My husband has a photograph of his father's father, standing very upright in his uniform, his skin a lighter shade than Swart Jong's and his high cheekbones revealing his Bushman ancestry.

I, too, have a photograph of my grandfather, Denholm Haden, standing next to his Spitfire, his pale eyes in a suntanned face. The same piercing blue eyes that attracted my grandmother's attention as she walked across a street in Carolina, Mpumalanga.

Did these two men ever meet in North Africa? Did they pass each other in the mess one day? Did my grandfather shout out an order to Henry Settler or ask him to shine his boots? How would their relationship have been different if they'd known they would share a great-great-grandson?

Sometimes, when I am very sad, I feel the presence of my ancestors, the women especially. I can sense them reaching down to comfort me.

Are they chatting amongst themselves now? Meeting in shared curiosity? 'Will it be a boy or girl? Whose eyes, ears, hair? Whose temperament? Will he look *old-fashioned*?'

Eventually my mind exhausts itself and I fall asleep.

In the morning practicalities take over. The ancestors have receded with the light that pours into the bedroom. I have regained some sanity and also my appetite, but I am not allowed to eat or drink anything before the operation. Just thinking about this makes my throat dry and my tummy rumble.

On the way to the hospital I keep checking my handbag as if I have left something crucial behind, like my passport.

We drive in silence, anxious about the next few hours. My husband sounds calm, but I know he is masking his own fear. He doesn't want to heighten my anxiety about the birth. But I know what his fears are.

In a hospital in Port Elizabeth his younger brother's son was stillborn. A perfectly healthy baby until the birth, he had been strangled by the umbilical cord. He was buried next to his granny, my mother-in-law, in a windswept graveyard on the outskirts of Port Elizabeth, overlooking the township where my husband grew up.

My husband and I have visited the grave, marked by a mound of earth and a simple wooden cross. Last year we took flowers for his mother. I looked down and imagined the tiny bones of my husband's stillborn nephew, buried at her feet. I was glad that he was with his granny for comfort.

⟲

At the hospital, we are directed to the maternity ward. A nurse takes us to the room I will be sharing with two others and hands me a gown to change into in preparation for the Caesar. Anxiety is briefly suspended as I enter another kind of time, travelling time, where normal life recedes. I am now in the departure lounge. There is no going back. A trolley arrives to wheel me down the corridor. My husband disappears and reappears in a fetching green theatre gown and fez-like cap. He looks handsome, I think to myself, like one of those doctors on *ER*. He smiles down at me and holds my hand as I make the last short journey into the operating theatre.

I am asked to sit on the edge of the bed and bend forward while the epidural is administered. When the anaesthetic takes effect the gynaecologist begins the incision. I can't see what's happening, as the gory bits are hidden behind a screen, but in a way that's worse. Trying to find ways to calm my nerves, I begin a running commentary to my husband. Amused, the obstetrician says to his assistant, 'We have a talker!' But it doesn't stop me. I can't do this in silence, and I continue to talk my way through the procedure like a reality cooking-show host.

'They are cutting through the layers of fat now . . . of which there aren't *that* many . . .'

Ignoring my nervous chatter, the obstetrician discusses a golfing dinner and his family's Christmas holiday. Then suddenly the room goes quiet. When he speaks again, his voice is tight, clipped, urgent. 'The umbilical cord is wrapped around the baby's neck.' I see the panic on my husband's face. It lasts a brief moment before our son is lifted free, red and screaming. The obstetrician had clamped and cut the cord three times to release him.

'It's lucky that you had a Caesar,' the anaesthetist tells me. 'The cord was very short.' Finally I am silenced. I have no regrets. My husband and I are tearful with relief and joy.

Our son is wrapped up and taken away, and I am moved to a trolley.

I look at my legs, which are like separate beings, completely numb.

When I am back in the ward, my husband fetches our son and lays him on my heart. He reaches out a tiny hand, his eyes screwed up tightly. He looks disgruntled and out of sorts. And I want to apologise to him.

Then I see the white band around his wrist, recording the time and date of his birth. 13/12/2004. I add the numbers up and there is something almost magical in the way they come back to 13.

On two family trees, another branch is drawn. The ancestors look down and smile. Samuel Morris Christopher Settler is written in black ink, underlined and bold. Such a long name for someone we will simply call Mo.

Water to Land

Elleke Boehmer

The town where I live is built on a floodplain and is often, winter and summer, awash with the unpredictable, soupy brown waters of the Thames. Even as I write this, the great river is flooding, lapping at the door of the house where I first learned what being a mother means. It seems appropriate somehow that, of the births of my two boys, of their transitions from watery embryo to dry land, the first took place in water, and the second slap-bang onto the ground, without ceremony.

My elder son, Thomas, who was always moving about rapidly in the womb, arrived like a silver fish in the hospital birthing pool, some time before his due date, in a rush. Sam, on the other hand, arrived exactly on time and wouldn't hear of his mum indulging herself with decorative props like monitors, beanbags or custom-made doula stools – certainly not a birthing pool. He was born fairly and squarely on dry land – in fact, on beige hospital lino – to a mother valiantly attempting to waddle to the same birthing pool, but caught short. In that difference, between a visitation and a fair-and-square arrival, lies the framework of this short narrative about their births.

While I hadn't expected Thomas to arrive in July, when I look back it's as if I was willing him to show up then. I'd been drinking quantities of raspberry leaf tea, walking miles, riding bikes down cobbled streets. For weeks I'd been ready for his coming. As labour began to establish itself, I phoned Val, my wise NHS midwife, to ask whether this really could be *it*. Sure enough, it was. Look up, she said, see the full moon in the sky. This was not a fanciful notion. More babies are born at the time of the full moon than at any other time; I don't know why. And so by the end of July, the second-last day in fact, there he was. A summer moon child.

'Turn around,' said Val, 'you have a baby boy.' I couldn't

believe it, though the pain had dropped right away. I'd been bobbing about in that milky-white water – water mixed in with the waters – for what felt like hours. I was starting to get used to it, almost. Turn around, she said. I edged away from the side, pivoted round. And whoosh, cupped in Val's hands, up through the water, came a scrawny, purple-white shape that she placed against my bent knees. Him. He took a small, almost imperceptible breath – his first, totally unassisted. There was no crying, no fuss. He opened his big eyes wide and, as if he'd seen it all before in some previous life, looked about him with a mild, unhurried curiosity.

This is what I thought. (I'll never forget this thought.) Looking at that face that was so new and fresh and untouched, that just a moment ago was still crumpled potential, not yet arrived, I thought, *OK, I get it*. I get death. Death might be easier than literature and our primal fear would have us expect. Now I know a tiny bit more of what it will be to die. It will be this eye-blink shift, not from not-life to life, as now, but in the reverse direction. I'll fear death less, I thought, because life is this quiet emergence from silence, and death presumably is a return to it. Death is ontologically impossible, say the philosophers. But being born, or indeed dying, that process of mysterious transition, is not: it is a living process.

In retrospect it seems crazy that death, non-being, was something I should confront at that moment, in that birthing pool. But it didn't seem bizarre at the time. It's what these experiences do to you, these portal experiences of birth, accompanying the dying, giving birth. For a moment you see everything in a clear and remote way. And then it's over. The new baby shifts himself on your knees. The water in the pool grows cold. The midwife announces that it's the end of her shift and she must be off. The new midwife ticks you off for bringing along no baby clothes whatsoever and only oversized nappies. You notice how loudly the clock on the wall has been ticking, all this time. Life moves itself on.

If I was hoping for a similar epiphany some years later with Sam, well, as someone in a Noel Streatfeild book used to say, I should have had another think coming. Sam announced himself around five p.m. on a Monday, as I was driving Thomas and a friend home from a swimming lesson. Ah, I thought, it's the due date, the baby may be on the way. Big twinge. So I dropped the friend at his house, then (going a bit more quickly now) dropped Thomas at another friend's, went home for my big green birthing ball – a very big twinge – and drove to the hospital. I'd opted for the hospital this second time because I was keen on having access to the pool once again.

I walked without a sideways glance past the Coke machine where five years and ten months before I'd stood braced as a massive contraction pulled through me. Here was the labour ward. An anonymous midwife stepped forward. Another very big twinge. I began to make noises about needing the birthing pool. But no. 'Another lady's in there,' she said. 'First come, first served.' I asked that the bed in the ward be moved to where I couldn't see it, so there'd be no temptation to use it and give birth on my back. Various midwives came and went, shifts ended. Huge twinge. Why didn't the woman in the birthing pool next door *hurry up*? I wanted that soothing water around me just about now. *Now*. But here was a complication. The baby's bouncing on his birth cord like a bungee jumper, they said, his amniotic sac won't break and let him free. This apparently wasn't great. There were frowns and covert looks. Still, I felt happy. To me this represented a chance to keep him safely inside until the birthing pool was available. My trainee midwife didn't agree. She shook her head and wouldn't meet my eye. She said that after this particular birth was successfully completed, she was entitled to her midwifery certificate. Evidently she wanted everything to unfold by the book.

By the book in this case meant the summoning of a second, more experienced midwife, ginger-haired and wielding a crochet hook, perhaps the buried signifier of brute reality – death – in this story. The crochet hook emerged, and was applied, and yanked, and then, with a greater whoosh than Thomas produced even in the water, a body-wrenching *yomp*, there was the baby: huge, pale, lying curled on the ground. My heart melted. Five years ago his brother and I sussed each other out before we cosied up. This one didn't wait. He opened one eye, decided work was over for the day and, cord still alive and pulsing, hunkered down on my funny, floppy stomach.

○

While Thomas's and Sam's birth elements may have been different, what firmly connected the two was, of course, their absolute physicality. Tiny, but infinitely present, warm-blooded, *embodied*, they tumbled full tilt, nothing caring, into the cerebral world I then inhabited. Yelling fit to burst, hiccuping for food until red in the face, they quickly disabused their mother of the idea that she might spend the foreseeable future reading *War and Peace* while idly jiggling the baby bouncer with her foot.

This new order of things was especially shocking the first time around. Within only a few days of Thomas's birth I was fully to confront the chasm I had just crossed, from writer-academic to mother (who, however, remained a writer-academic). I was walking down High Street carrying baby in baby carrier, plus changing bag, shawl and other baby paraphernalia, when I passed a former student of mine, a young woman sociable and friendly by nature. And she did not *see* me. She passed within inches; she noticed, she certainly did notice, a certain frowsy mother shape walking gingerly past (pelvis still righting itself some three days after the birth), but she did not recognise in that shape the person she had known, her tutor. To her, babies and the scholarly world were so thoroughly irreconcilable as to cancel each other out, and that paradox made me invisible.

There were other things, too, that I hadn't expected before being pregnant. I was to discover that the temperament of a child suggests itself a while before the birth, and is then, you could say, announced at the delivery. Previously a believer in nurture over nature, I was more than surprised by this. Thomas, fittingly, has continued in his life to be a maelstrom of energy and sensitivity, as if his impatience to leave the womb had been a matter of personal urgency. Sam's very unceremonious, terrestrial arrival is similarly consistent with a child who is fiercely set in his ways, tenacious, decisive, grounded.

From water to land: one child all liquidity, the other earthed. And their mother (all mothers?) constantly trying to reconcile their elements, ever in motion between them.

A Thousand Births

Phillippa Yaa de Villiers

I think maybe what I wanted and what I want
is to remember,
that's all,
remember my story clearly.
My mind is a hand
reaching out to trace
the features of a forgotten face.[1]

Being adopted is like being born a thousand times, your identity displaced in continually re-imagined scenes of your origins. Discovering that the story you've grown up with and trusted is false is like being informed that you've been living under an assumed name. Like a character in a spy thriller, you enter the realm of fiction.

My father sat down with me on Bakoven beach on a cold winter afternoon in 1982. I was twenty years old. I remember the sound of the waves on the rocks punctuating his words. 'Phillippa, you are going places where your mother and I cannot follow. We won't be able to protect you.'

'What do you mean?' I asked, puzzled. 'Almost everyone I know is being followed by the security police. It's no big deal.'

He said, 'But, you see, you are not like your friends. You are not white. Your birth mother is a white Australian. Your biological father is possibly of Aboriginal extraction, we're not sure.'

I watched a dark wall of water shattering on the rocks. In the depths between the truth I had known and this new reality, I trod water, trying not to drown. Why did my mother give me up for adoption? And why in apartheid-era South Africa? I struggled to fathom the reasons.

---

1 Extract from 'Wanting', in *Taller than Buildings* (self-published, December 2006).

Growing up, I used to joke that I had hatched from an egg, or that, like baby Superman, a cherub in a Kryptonite capsule, I had been randomly hurled to earth. In the years that followed that cold afternoon on Bakoven beach, I found other ways of fictionalising myself, as I built a career in scriptwriting and performing. I conjured and reconjured my origins in the poems and stories I wrote, and in the scripts I acted out on stage. Freedom lay in becoming someone else. I could imagine countless characters, mimic their accents, take on their physicality, but my own being was an enigma. I couldn't say what I really looked like or, often, how I felt. I was invisible to myself. Because who was I, exactly? Where did I come from?

At some level I knew that I would only ever find solace and stability in my real story, and so I began to search for whatever facts I could find.

I discovered my biological parents in the same year that I conceived my son. My mother was still living in Australia. My father, it turned out, was of Ghanaian origin, but was by now a naturalised Australian. In retrospect, it was as if I had to find them before I myself could become a parent. It was the beginning of my initiation into the ranks of humanity – our muscle and gristle, bone and blood. Without close family ties, I had been unique – for some, enviably – yet alienated, alone, obdurately singular. I didn't know what it felt like to be bound irrevocably to somebody. People with natural parents seemed to live in a perfect world, while I didn't ever feel fully human. This recovery of my bloodline, which would culminate in the birth of my own child, was to free me from years of self-doubt and depression.

But it was still early days, and as the date of my son's birth approached, I began to worry. Would I abandon my baby, turn my face to the wall and refuse to touch him, as my birth mother had done? The midwife was reassuring: 'You must separate your experience from your son's – he has a different life. He is being born into new, separate circumstances.' Comforting as these words were on one level, the word 'separate' sliced into me.

I chose to give birth at home without pain medication.

My friends laughed and cajoled me. 'Come on, the drugs are completely safe – thousands of healthy babies are born and their mothers are spared the agony of childbirth. Anyway, you were never one to say no to drugs.' It was true. During my late teens and early twenties I had experimented with various mind-altering substances. Yet I wanted to be wide awake and present for every second of my labour. I wanted to be able to tell my son every detail.

○

My son, on the night you started your journey into the world, the West African Muslims who had made a mosque of the house behind ours were holding an all-night service. Voices rose out of the darkness like sparks from a fire. It was winter in Johannesburg, dry and freezing.

Earlier in the evening, your dad and I had shared a pizza with friends. It was the final meeting of our creative-writing work group. I had all kinds of plans for my future writing life. I was writing-fit, excited about the television series I was busy developing, feeling my creative powers in full swing.

Later, as we lay in bed, I didn't connect the bump in my belly with the cramps that chased me out from beneath the warm covers to the toilet three times, until your dad gently rubbed my belly. 'Maybe you shouldn't have had that pizza?' he asked. Only then did the thought cross my mind, like an uncertain comic walking on stage in front of a hostile audience. 'I don't think it's the pizza,' I said.

Your dad put on one of our favourite CDs, The Buena Vista Social Club, and lit some candles. I hesitated before calling one of the two midwives who were going to deliver you. But another contraction had me punching out the numbers.

'Take a Panado,' she told me. 'They don't cross the placental barrier. Try to rest. Phone me in the morning if you're still sore.'

Your dad paced gleefully up and down. Fifteen minutes passed, during which the pains intensified and I started to feel restless. He sat down, watching me. I watched his expression turn. 'So now what do we do?' he asked. 'I don't know,' I said. 'Aren't you supposed to boil some water?'

We used the boiling water for tea, not for the delivery. And we sat there for what seemed like hours listening to the old Cubans singing their soothing songs, stories of love and regret born out of a lifetime's experience.

Your dad's hands rubbed encouragement into my back. I remember the feeling of his touch growing fainter and fainter. I looked around. He had fallen asleep. I realised that waking him would be pointless. I would have to do this part alone. He had done his share, and he would help again later.

I squatted, I walked, I pressed my back hard against the wall and wiggled my pelvis. I listened to the radio and the caterwauling of mating cats in the darkness outside. I danced. I ran a hot bath and soaked in it. But I couldn't escape the relentless contractions. I lost all sense of time. The past seemed somewhere very far below the present.

At six a.m. I let go of my manners and phoned the midwife again. 'Come here now. Please.' Then I got back into the bath. Your dad had woken up and brought me a cup of tea.

'I suppose you don't really want to hear a joke?' he asked me.

'I do, I do, yes, please make me laugh!' I begged. Our laughter came like the early morning sun in the blue winter sky.

The midwives arrived to deliver you. They worked as a pair, like many of my favourite acts: Popeye and Olive Oyl, Thelma and Louise, Wallace and Gromit. They complemented each other visually and in their conversational style. One was tall and blonde, the other short. One was dreamy and diplomatic, the other firm and practical. Both were easy to talk to, with a fine sense of humour.

I was consumed with restlessness and couldn't work out how to settle. So I paced the house naked, feeling absurd, while the midwives started preparing the bedroom for the birth, like altar servers getting the church ready for a service.

Suddenly their cheery purposefulness infuriated me. I had had enough. I strode to the kitchen, ready to quit. 'I'm sick of this now,' I snapped. 'I'm not doing this any more.' Your dad was quite thrown by this, and reminded me that I didn't really have a choice. The obviousness of this fact annoyed me even more. I sat stubbornly at the kitchen table, tears streaming down my face. The midwives came and sat with us. 'I don't want to have a baby,' I wept. 'I'm not ready for the responsibility.' They ignored this and calmly asked me what I was going to call you.

'I want to call him Nestor, after the butler in the Tintin books, but he won't have it.' I nodded savagely at your dad. Nobody laughed. (Since then I have had the greatest respect for people who know how to treat a person who is being ridiculous. I respect their compassion, their indulgence, their patience and love.)

'Shall we go to the bedroom?' the short midwife asked. The door to the bedroom was the port where I would have to dock, releasing my passenger. But I wasn't ready. I liked having you on board. You made no demands, swam the length of my belly kicking gently, were clever and gentle and perfect inside there. Outside in the profane world, what would become of that perfection?

Although it was obviously pointless to resist, my mind refused to cross the threshold.

Time passed, I don't know how long, and I started to see images of openings – doors, tunnels, windows, caves, open to the weather. I looked at the bedroom door, and somewhere in me another door opened. I held on to the image; it was all I had. 'I'm ready now,' I said, as I lay on the bed.

And there you were. I looked into your small face. The bluish cord led out of your abdomen somewhere into the heart of me. Your head, squeezed into a cone shape by the exertion of birth, seemed to emphasise the look of gentle puzzlement on your face. You seemed to be thinking, 'Who are you, and what are you doing here?'

Your name came out of my mouth as if it had always lain there, waiting to be called: Felix.

You were my first blood relative – now I knew how it felt. Profound, yet blessedly ordinary. And my adoptive family and friends were even more beloved because, as I was to realise, reality is not in the blood. It's in the loving. I'd never have known this if it weren't for you. You gave me kinship and a mirror.

When you were eight months old, I saw your grandparents for the first time. Your grandfather – a perfect stranger with a nose identical to mine – met us at the airport. He immediately took you from me and hugged you, closing the broken circle. We were home – sort of. My Australian birth mother arranged a barbecue to celebrate our arrival, and my sister and I tried hard not to stare at each other, mesmerised as we were by the double mirror of our chins, our eyes, our gaze. I was so happy to discover our resemblances, but sad, too, to feel the separateness of our lives.

But you and I had each other.

My son, we are born with a story and the story contains the world. Your story contained my story tangled up inside it, just as you were tangled up inside me. This is our story. Your birth washed us up on to a new shore.

> Tonight my son, my favourite poem,
> shares my bed. His gentle snores,
> like footprints on the night.
>
> He is upside down. What dream
> is holding him
> by the ankle?[2]

---

2 Extract from 'Origin', 2007 (unpublished).

Queen Charlotte's Child

Andrew Weeks

We were playing it safe. Yet Zoë, our first-born, died at birth in England's oldest maternity unit – *one of the best* – in the leafy suburb of W6, London, The Greatest City on Earth. She did not start breathing, and her heart stopped for twenty minutes or more. Time had stopped, too. Perhaps she was never technically, clinically dead, but it was a death to me. Even if she lived, it seemed the best – or worst – we could hope for was a brain-dead baby.

Our child's first taste was not sweet mother's milk. It was intravenous morphine and the tang of a cold steel instrument – like a high-tech tent peg – rammed deep into her gagging throat.

In those first fluorescent seconds, I noticed that Zoë had my stubborn grandmother's face. Her tiny naked yellow body convulsed and thrashed like an insect impaled on a pin. A livid patch of raspberry pulsed dead centre in her forehead like a third eye. Lucky for her. I stood beside the bed and watched and felt freeze-dried.

The full facts of the story are no longer important. No doctor could provide a medical explanation for what happened. Only now, with a decade's hindsight, do my fragmentary impressions form some kind of coherent narrative.

I remember my partner, Penny, and me attending antenatal classes in north London. We sit cross-legged on the floor drinking chai, watching films of Amazonians squatting briefly to give birth. Penny enjoys a healthy full-term pregnancy. She runs a few days overdue. There's an instruction to book an induction.

Then, finally, on the eve of hospital admission, a slow start. We're told to go home at 1 cm at one a.m. in pissing rain. We come back at four p.m. No bed available yet. A coffee room with ratty sofas and a small fuzzy TV. A large porter snores in the corner. Penny weeps. I implore nurses to do something. We only get a room when we threaten to go to St Mary's Paddington. Penny has a bath. We are assigned an uninterested pimply young midwife. Lesley, I think. Seven p.m., 2 cm. Cigarettes in the car park. Penny paces corridors, climbs stairs and rides lifts, moaning. Eleven p.m., 2 cm. We're given a late diagnosis of *occipital posterior presentation*, in which mother's and child's vertebrae rub painfully against each other, slowing labour. Too late to be helpful. Then a shot of accelerator hormone. A long night of spine-grinding, unproductive labour, which assiduous aromatherapy and acupuncture fail to relieve.

A change of shift at dawn. A fresh midwife – a buxom, cheerful Irishwoman named Bella. A change of tactics, too, from acupuncture needles to the epidural variety. I fixate on the tiny margin of error, and the unthinkable consequences of a cock-up. I watch a needle the width of a screwdriver being driven into precisely the right gap in Penny's heaving backbone, and want to hug the earnest, sweating anaesthetist. A cunning dispenser is taped to Penny's shoulder. Relief on tap. Relief all round. Penny has a cup of tea, a short stroll and a catnap, before the final push. I drag deeply at the gas and air mask, which Penny does not want, and become light-headed. A stern, bespectacled specialist makes a fleeting appearance during his rounds, noting a few initial, though minor, signs of foetal distress. There's now some sense of urgency, and an ultimatum (twenty minutes?), punctuated by the words *episiotomy* and *forceps. Or else an emergency Caesar*. Bella's scalpel slices sickeningly through vaginal muscle. Our baby's wrinkled waxy scalp crowns . . .

Followed by a chaotic, lurching tableau of searing events and impressions. As the child is delivered, the delivery suite and assembled personnel are hosed with shocking, poppy-red blood. (This is later discovered to have been the result of the umbilical cord suddenly rupturing, like a burst bicycle tube, something I have never heard of happening to anyone else.)[1] There is more

---

1 After writing this story, I did some research on the Internet, and discovered synopses

urgency, though no visible panic, not yet, not to me. White backs hunch over the newborn, held down on a table while the tent peg keeps her throat open. A tube sucks the sticky black foetal shit, like so much toxic creosote, from her lungs. I croak *Is she OK?* and am offered reassuring, backhanded blandnesses. *Meconium, see it all the time, she'll be fine.* Still the baby does not breathe, or cry. Is this normal? I've never seen a baby born before. An oxygen tube is stuffed down her gullet. Still she shows no sign of breathing. I get further, less convincing, versions of *Don't worry, under control* from an ashen-faced young medic. Blood congeals on the floor. The placenta must have been delivered. We feel locked out. I try to comfort Penny, lying spent and forgotten on the steel bed. I can't meet her eyes. There is a grim inevitability to all this. Then someone says *heart failure*. Or *cardiac arrest*. Either way, it meant the same thing.

Several doctors, perhaps four or five, mill around in starchy, white-coated confusion. This is not the stuff from which textbooks are scripted. Someone tries ineffectually to pump this tiny creature's chest, but he's already lost hope. Rising voices, quickening. There's no longer any pretence of being in control. We're at the accident scene of a birth gone awfully awry. Help. A call of *Intensive Care!* punctures the panic.

Then an angel, called to resurrect my daughter, bursts through the theatre's swing-doors. She's a blonde, no-nonsense Australian trauma nurse in a green surgical smock, who looks no more than twenty. She ignores the laws of hospital hierarchies, giving crisp instructions, like someone ordering vital cocktails above the commotion of a busy Soho bar. *Adrenaline! Morphine! Glucose drip!* The dithering doctors humbly obey. She massages Zoë's little sternum and calmly begins to work her alchemy. I imagine I see a pink flush slowly infuse the limp form on the table, or perhaps not. Orderlies wheel in a perspex-covered incubator,

---

of articles from two medical journals (one French, one German) about a rare condition referred to as *spontaneous umbilical cord haematoma*, which occurs in less than 1 in 5 500 births, a rate of 0.018 per cent. The French article stated: 'Umbilical cord haematomas are usually responsible for severe foetal distress or death.' The German article stated: 'A haematoma of the umbilical cord is frequently fatal for the foetus.'

like a space-age cake trolley. Our prone child is plugged in and wheeled out, a drip swinging above her. If she breathes, it's only by the grace of an oxygen canister nestled like a bomb beneath the trolley. It's forty-five minutes since her delivery at 11:40 a.m. on Wednesday, 3 December 1997.

We are alone, tear-streaked and stunned. Some time later, the senior consultant obstetrician on duty comes into the room. Her stony face is moving. She tells us she cannot tell us anything. Not whether our baby is alive, or dead, or something in-between. She takes five minutes to do a shoddy job stitching Penny together again. Left alone once more, I mumble some unforgivable things to Penny about *not being able to let go.* Otherwise we don't talk. We are offered NHS tea and soggy biscuits. The possibilities must have jostled for space inside my skull, but I recall only blankness. Perhaps I had a cigarette downstairs. We wait for three hours, and several more ages. A person puts her head around the door. Maybe it's Bella. *She's alive.* This should be good news, but does not sound like it. We are taken, in a trembling fog, down to Intensive Care two floors below.

We see Zoë inside her bubble, and are flooded by a sense of cautious relief. Our child is alive and fighting, trying to remove needles from her forearm and tubes from her nostrils, and shaking her head. She looks determined to free herself from this medical bondage. We fall headlong in love with her gutsy spirit, but a nagging, lurking fear stifles any premature celebration.

Twenty-four hours after her birth, Zoë starts breastfeeding. She rapidly moves out of danger and into the affections of the ICU staff. She has shrugged off death before being truly alive. After three days she comes home and I return to a stressful new job in the City. We effusively thank and praise the hospital medics. We never see the Australian nurse again. Several weeks and many specialist appointments later, Zoë's milestones seem normal. An ECG scan reveals some damage to the plastic 'white matter' at the brain's periphery, but soft-spoken Dr Azzopardi explains that this is probably reversible, because the grey matter looks intact. The prognosis is optimistic. Which it proves, so far (so good), to have been. Six weeks later, we name our child Zoë

(Greek for 'life'), before a Hammersmith registrar.

Months after that, perhaps a year or two before the distinctive red-brick of Queen Charlotte's Hospital[2] was demolished to make way for council housing, I made a copy of the medical records of the birth, and archived the bulging file in the attic unread. Penny and I have since separated.

---

2 Queen Charlotte's Maternity Hospital was named after Duchess Sophia Charlotte of Mecklenburg-Strelitz, King George III's queen, who had fifteen children. Because of her 'mulatto' features, Charlotte is thought by some to have had African ancestry. The southern African flower *Strelitzia reginae* (in bloom outside my window in Cape Town as I write) was also named after Queen Charlotte.

The Birth of a Son

Sindiwe Magona

I began borrowing Nomvuyo Ngcelwane's overall in the fifth
month of my pregnancy. I had ballooned and had *nothing* to
wear. Nomvuyo, a friend and neighbour, had given birth to her
son a month before, the same month my husband had walked
out, leaving me pregnant and penniless, with two little girls. It
was amazing, the creativity that desperation lent me, aged only
twenty-three. Nomvuyo had used that overall as a maternity
dress, but now I needed it more than she did – unless I was
to parade myself naked and pregnant to Somerset Hospital's
prenatal clinic.

Nomvuyo was (and still is) a stylish lady. How lucky for me!
To this day I have a vivid picture in my mind of that overall:
bright pink with a black lace collar. I *should* remember it, too!
For four solid months, I wore it every Friday, for my visits to the
prenatal clinic. The borrowing became a standing arrangement.

One Thursday afternoon in my ninth month, as had become
customary, I sent a child to ask Nomvuyo if I might borrow her
overall. Early the next morning, the last Friday in September, I
set off for Nyanga Station. There I bought a third-class return
ticket to town. The meagre sum of money at my disposal from
selling *skaapkop*[1] would not extend to first-class fares (or indeed
second-class either!). When the train arrived, I pushed my way
in with the rest of the folk. At that time of morning, taking
public transport was quite an ordeal. People were in a rush
trying to get to work, most of them already late. They would
jostle and shove to secure a seat on the overcrowded trains. In
such a situation, one could hardly expect to be noticed, let alone
be given special attention or kindness. So, on that particular
Friday, I pushed like everyone else into the carriage packed with

---

1 'Sheep heads'.

106

the working poor, like human sardines.

'Normal' people took buses from Cape Town to Green Point. There was nothing normal about my situation. I took 'CA 10'. In other words, I walked. (CA is the registration prefix for cars in Cape Town, and 10 refers to the number of toes on two feet.) Who could afford the luxury of a bus ride? Not me. In due course, I got my pregnant self to the hospital, a long time after the women I had seen on the train earlier that morning, who had taken the bus. I joined the seemingly endless queue. And, after the usual routine – the endless wait and shuffling from hall to hall – I eventually landed at the doctor's station, for the examination.

'Mama,' said he, excitedly, 'I think we have twins here!'

I do not look it, but I am tough as nails. That I did not have a heart attack right then and there attests to that fact. I have nothing against twins. When I was growing up, being the mother of twins was one of my romantic notions, probably because I come from a family singularly lacking in multiple births of any kind. I remember how I would wistfully say, 'Oh, I hope I will have three sets of twins when I grow up!' I even knew the gender I wanted – and in what order. Something must have warned me that these twins would be hard work, because I wanted the boys last: girls, girls, then boys. See, by the time I had the third set, I would need a lot of help. Well, I'd had two girls, albeit single births. Would it be a question of third time lucky?

Well, when the man in his white jacket said those words, my heart leapt up and caught in my throat, especially when he added, 'And they want to come out – today, I think!' *Today?* This was only the last week of October. I was supposed to have another three weeks or so. How could such a thing happen? I was hardly prepared for the single baby I was expecting in three weeks' time. I was not working. And not being a citizen of the country, as the government of the time saw it, I was not eligible for any public assistance. As matters stood, the sum total of this baby's layette was two vests, two nighties, six napkins, one receiving blanket and a ninety-nine-cent shawl. This last item was bought not for beauty, but to disguise the absence of a real, woollen, baby blanket. Its price illustrates that all the items were chosen for one reason and one reason only: they were the cheapest I could find. But if this not so much scanty as downright inadequate layette was cause for concern for one infant, how could it possibly be sufficient for twins?

'I'm sending you for an X-ray,' the doctor announced triumphantly as he handed me my folder and pointed the way to the X-ray wing of the hospital. He wanted to verify his suspicion.

I fought back tears. 'Please, God!' I prayed. 'Don't answer my prayer now. Not like this.' It had suddenly occurred to me that God might find it funny to answer the stupid wish I'd so carelessly expressed as a child.

The bright sunlight did nothing to cheer me up as I crossed the courtyard on my way to the X-ray block, the folder in my hand heavier than sin. What would I do if it were twins? Where would I get the clothes for two babies, when I didn't have enough for one? What would they eat, for surely my milk would not be enough for two? 'Please, God, don't let it be twins,' I pleaded. I doubt I have ever been more fervent in prayer. The double blessing I had yearned for in my youthful ignorance of the harsh realities of life would have been a double curse to me just then.

As luck would have it, the X-ray showed it was a false alarm. However, something was amiss all right. The baby was in a breech position, which threatened to split open the weakened, twice-opened Caesarean scar on my belly. So, no sooner was I relieved of the anxiety that I was about to give birth to twins than I was plunged into another tizzy. Now the hospital wanted to send me by ambulance, at once, to Groote Schuur Hospital. I was told that the baby was to be delivered the next day. But why Groote Schuur, I wondered? The reason for the transfer had not been explained to me, and it did not occur to me that I could ask. We were people who did not question authority, and august persons like doctors, it seemed, never explained things to their patients. 'We're sending you to Groote Schuur, by ambulance,' I was told.

But that was just impossible, not doable, in my case. At home I was the resident adult, not only for my two young daughters, but for my four younger siblings. Mama had gone to Tsolo in the Eastern Cape to be at her father's deathbed. Tata was away at sea, on the fishing trawlers going to Tristan da Cunha, and wouldn't be back till Christmas week. I was in charge of the household. Therefore, I couldn't just up and go to Groote Schuur, or any other place, for that matter. I had to make arrangements first.

Although the oldest of these children was sixteen, I couldn't just leave them alone. I had to make sure that there would be food to eat while I was away and an adult eye watching over them. Of course, this was all something that could have been done by phone anywhere else in the world. Not in South Africa, not at that time – for Africans, anyway. There were no telephones in the houses of the townships. One had to have a very good reason to be allowed to apply for a phone, such as a heart problem or some similarly critical condition. Phones were not to be had simply for the sake of having them. They were in the same category as inside toilets, hot water and electricity – 'luxuries' not available in the townships.

I explained as much to the doctor and the nurses. I gave my word that I would not sleep in Gugulethu, but go to Groote Schuur that very same day. Back home I hastily made the necessary arrangements. I asked a relative, who lived on the same street, to keep an eye on the children, left what little money I had with her, gave numerous instructions to my siblings and alerted an aunt to the situation. She kindly agreed to come to the house every night until my return. Lastly, I sent a telegram to my husband. To this day I don't know why I bothered. What could I have expected from a man who had left me four months ago and had not given us a cent by way of support since? At that time, however, it seemed the right thing to do – to tell a man that his child was about to be born.

I did all I had to do, then made my way to Groote Schuur Hospital as I had promised. I was pregnant. I was destitute. Yet I was definitely not suicidal. It was crystal clear in my mind that

I would be endangering my life and the life of the unborn child if I did not do as the doctor had ordered. So, I did exactly that.

Although I got to the hospital just in time for supper, it was only to find I would be put on a 'nil per mouth' restriction for the rest of that night. This was done in preparation for going to theatre the next morning. Thus, my son was born on 28 October, a Saturday morning – four months, one week and five days after his father had abandoned the family. But the matron at Groote Schuur Hospital wouldn't believe it if she read this today.

Ordinarily, one doesn't get a visit from the matron, but I did. That lady was deeply impressed that my loving husband had called the hospital, distraught that he could not be by my side at this difficult time.

'Is your husband away on duty, Mama?' the matron enquired. Weakly, I nodded.

To this day, I cannot say whether I aided and abetted my husband's deceit because of embarrassment or out of sheer stupidity. Why didn't I just blurt it out: 'That lying so-and-so! What duty? He left me, pregnant and with two little ones, in June! What's more, he has not sent us a lousy cent!' No, I didn't say any of that. I said nothing at all. Just nodded – like the fool I was. The fool my husband knew I was. That knowledge, that certainty, is the only thing that could have given him the gall to do what he did – call the hospital and lie shamelessly. He certainly knew me. I was not about to confess when all those women in the ward would hear me tell the matron the truth, my shame. Because that is what I felt then, what I believed, that the shame was mine. Don't ask me how I could have been so stupid. A man abandons his wife and children – and it is the wife who has a sense of shame! Not the man, oh no! But then, I am a product of my time, of the people of whom I am a part. Then, as now, the woman was humiliated in such circumstances. *Idikazi*, she is labelled from there on. *Idikazi* is 'a husbandless woman of marriageable age', according to the dictionary. The same authority assures us that this is 'a term of reproach'. At the tender age of twenty-three, I had become such a woman.

You should have seen the matron's eyes when, later the same

day, an enormous bouquet of flowers arrived for me. Yes, from my dear husband. So huge and ornate was the arrangement of flowers that word spread like a *veld* fire and nurses, on day and on night duty, came to ooh and aah over them. I don't mind telling you, those flowers were something to behold. Not one of the nurses could have suspected that the father who sent such a bouquet had not bothered to give a cent towards the purchase of even one napkin for his baby. I bet anyone anything that the price of those flowers far exceeded the amount I had paid for my baby's layette in its miserly totality.

The only cause for joy throughout my stay in hospital, about a week or so, was that I had given birth to a bouncing, eight-pound, eight-ounce boy. My baby was perfect. All his organs were exactly where they were supposed to be. There were precisely the number of fingers and toes there were supposed to be – in perfect proportion. I was ecstatic. Worries about clothing and feeding him dimmed, for the moment.

But I was not allowed to be completely happy and carefree. The woman in the bed next to mine, also mother to a son, could neither read nor write. Neither could her husband. The two were totally illiterate, and they signed by making an X. I know because I had to translate for them when they had to consent to her undergoing an operation. She'd also delivered by Caesarean section.

The woman's husband came to visit her every evening. This was a reminder to me of my husband's absence, of his betrayal and neglect. Compared to my neighbour, I was highly educated. I boasted a Junior Certificate academic qualification and a two-year Higher Primary Teachers' Certificate. I was a qualified teacher. But that was not the only humiliation I suffered – I, who thought of herself as better, by virtue of her education! When this woman was discharged from hospital, her husband was waiting with a hired car for his wife and newborn son. I, on the other hand, had to find my way home unsupported, by bus.

I am a slow learner. I did not go as soon as we were discharged in the morning. Oh no, I waited for someone to come and help me carry this big baby. Remember, I had a fresh scar, and I knew that one had to be very careful not to carry too much weight. My sister-in-law was coming to help me get home. My mother was still on her way back from Tsolo. She had left as soon as the news had reached her that I was in hospital.

I waited and waited, sitting on a chair by someone else's bed, as my bed had long since been allocated to another patient. When lunch was served, I realised that I had not only lost my bed, but I had no right to a plate of food either. Discharged, I no longer had any claim on the services provided by the hospital. It seemed odd to me, not to say inhospitable, that the same hospital that had cared for me and my son should, at the stroke of a pen, be so uncaring. Embarrassment drove me out of that ward. I was not going to sit there and watch the other patients eating. Other patients? I was no longer a patient. The only reason I was still there was that no one had come to fetch me.

Groote Schuur lies on the hip of a mountain, which is to say, it is on an incline, high up from the road. All the way down that long slope, each step I took pulled at the taut stitches in my midriff, and tears streamed down my cheeks. These were not just tears of pain; they were tears of mortification. I felt as unwanted as trash. I had never hated my husband before. I hated him then. With all my heart, I hated him. We would never be divorced, legally; but in my heart, that is when I divorced him.

Finally, exhausted, I reached the Main Road. Being a Sunday, I had a long wait for the bus. When it finally came, it was a double-decker. This was the time of segregated seating on buses: whites downstairs, and non-whites upstairs. I must have looked wretched enough that several people immediately offered me a seat – downstairs. I gratefully accepted. I got off in Claremont, then stood in another queue for another bus. This time to Gugulethu, with my brand-new baby boy – Sandile Soyiso.

Each in Its Own Way

Marita van der Vyver

My teenage son stumbles sleepily into our kitchen and blinks in astonishment when he hears the sounds being broadcast by the battered old radio next to the stove. He turns to me as the peculiar panting and increasingly high-pitched moaning form a crescendo.

'Ma, are you listening to *porn*?'

'No, Daniel,' I answer. 'I'm listening to someone giving birth.' Which, admittedly, does sound rather like someone having really great sex.

This happened early one morning last week. A reporter from a major French radio station had spent a night in a maternity ward and was now offering millions of listeners this moving recording of a birth reaching its climax. And despite the fact that I had seen similar scenes acted out countless times on screen, by actresses with varying degrees of talent, there was something particularly touching about this auditory birth experience. Mainly because it was not acted; it was real. And since the action was invisible, left to each listener's imagination, it lost some of its uniqueness and acquired a universal quality.

I'm sure any listener who had ever given birth, or watched a loved one giving birth, couldn't help identifying with the panting, the moaning and, finally, those ecstatic sobs of relief. My arms were covered in goose pimples.

I didn't try to explain any of this to my bemused sixteen-year-old son – if he's fortunate enough to become a father one day, he'll understand. But as I ate my breakfast cereal, my thoughts drifted to Tolstoy's famous statement about universality and uniqueness, that unforgettable opening sentence of *Anna Karenina*: *All happy families are alike; each unhappy family is unhappy in its own way.* Could the same comfortable blanket of generalisation possibly be thrown over the experience of giving birth? Could we say that all happy births are alike, but each unhappy birth is unhappy in its own way?

Yes, I thought, *of course*. And then, *No, of course not*.

I should be able to answer the question without waffling. I've given birth three times, to children from three different fathers from three different cultures and language groups, in two countries, on two continents. So I suppose I can say without fear of contradiction that my experience is more varied than that of most mothers.

The first birth was probably the most traumatic experience of my life. Owing to medical negligence, the baby was born with severe brain damage. The doctor failed to arrive after the nurse had phoned to tell him that I was fully dilated, and the nursing staff, instead of acting on the baby's signs of distress, preferred to wait. They told me to be patient, to close my legs, not to push. I listened to them, of course, not realising that, in this drawn-out waiting period, the child was being deprived of oxygen. By the time the doctor got there, the damage was done. My son Ian was blind and deaf, and would never be able to walk or talk or even swallow food. He spent nearly all of his miserable life in hospital, constantly battling infections of the respiratory system, and died shortly before his first birthday.

For the next two births I insisted on a Caesarean section to ensure that the baby would get out as quickly as possible, with as little risk of damage as possible. Those were probably the two most exhilarating, profound experiences of my life.

A while ago I described the devastating experience of my first child's birth in fictional form. It took me a decade and a half to build up enough courage to do it, to go back there and write a short story about it.[1] The process of writing brought me a measure of peace, if not closure. *Closure* is one of those trendy therapeutic terms flung around to cover infinitely intricate emotional processes. In my personal experience, certain holes never close. You just learn to watch out for them, tread carefully

1 The story, 'Circular Flight', can be read in *Short Circuits* by Marita van der Vyver (Cape Town: Tafelberg, 2005).

around them, for the rest of your life.

The two 'happy births' did more to help me live with that hole than any amount of therapy and writing and creativity ever could. Yet even these births – despite all the obvious similarities, the same method, the same sounds, the same sensations – were happy in unique ways.

One consequence of my traumatic birth experience was that I lost my belief that nowadays birth is easy and safe and clean, almost comfortable. Once you have seen how horribly wrong a modern birth can go, you realise that birth is bloody and messy and sometimes life-threatening, for both baby and mother. Certainly not comfortable, and not always safe.

I was tormented by this knowledge when I became pregnant again. It happened barely a year after the death of my first-born – as it often does, I would later learn. It seemed that my body's only defence against the shock of a defective birth was to go into a kind of reproductive overdrive. A frenzy of fertility, whether I wanted it or not. I certainly didn't plan another pregnancy quite so soon. One of the sad results of my child's death was that my marriage had disintegrated. (Another frequent occurrence after the loss of a child, as I would also learn.) A year later I was divorced and found myself husbandless, homeless, jobless – and pregnant.

Emotionally I was far too dazed and confused to venture into another long-term romantic relationship, so when I learnt I was pregnant, I chose what I then regarded as the easy option. I would fly solo, I decided. I would become a single mother.

Looking back, I could say many things about single motherhood, but one thing I would never say is that it's an *easy* option. If I'd known then what I know now, I might not have done it. My ignorance was a blessing. The result, after all, is this tall teenage son whom I adore – even though he suspects his middle-aged mother of listening to porn on the kitchen radio. I watch him buttering his toast while I pour myself a cup of coffee. Sixteen years down the line I still sometimes find it hard to believe that this one made it.

I planned his birth like a military operation, down to the

last detail. This time there would be a paediatrician with me in the labour ward to care for the baby from its first breath. I also felt far better prepared myself, having done this before. I told myself I would know if things were going wrong – I would demand urgent action, I would scream and shout. I wouldn't just lie there, foolishly trusting modern medicine as I had done the first time.

And this time I had my mother with me. It made all the difference, not only because she was a qualified nursing sister with solid obstetric experience, but because she was my mother. It's only when we become mothers ourselves that we really appreciate our mothers. This is one of the lessons I'd learnt when my first son was born.

During that first birth, my sister was far away in England, where her husband was studying, my brother was surfing somewhere along the Cape coast and my parents were patiently waiting for news at their home in Cape Town. All of us so stupidly sure that all would be well. When I went into labour the second time, the scenario was completely different. My sister, who was then living in Namibia, walked unannounced into the maternity ward in Cape Town. 'I tried waiting at home,' she explained with some embarrassment, 'but I was such a nervous wreck that my husband booked me a seat on the first plane.' My brother promptly dropped his surfboard and drove to the hospital, where he hung around for hours. My child's father was also there, accompanied by his mother for moral support. And my mother held my hand throughout the epidural Caesarean.

The only missing person was my father – but then he'd also missed his own children's births. He belonged to an age where birth was women's work and men waited in the wings, anxiously smoking and afterwards buying drinks for complete strangers in the nearest bar. Yet the moment my mother phoned to tell him that he could now call himself the proud grandfather of a perfect baby boy, he jumped into his car to join the rest of the family celebrating around my hospital bed.

His elation was undoubtedly heightened by the fact that the newborn was a boy – a huge surprise to all of us, because according to two ultrasound scans this one was supposed to be a girl. Psychologically I'd been preparing myself for a girl. True, I hadn't made any practical preparations – as in knitting pink booties or buying frilly dresses – but that was simply another consequence of the previous disastrous experience. For the first baby everything had been ready weeks in advance: the clothes, the equipment, the stroller, the cot . . . and then I'd had to come home without the baby. Giving away all these unnecessary items had been like biting off chunks of my own flesh. This time I preferred to be unprepared for the event.

Because in spite of everything – the meticulous planning, the constant medical supervision throughout the pregnancy, the comforting presence of my mother during labour – in spite of all this, I hadn't *really* been able to believe that this time the baby would be fine.

I hadn't even bought a carrycot for the child, which meant that Daniel had to spend his first few nights at home sleeping in a drawer. My father was terribly upset that his namesake and only grandchild should be treated in such an undignified way – until I reminded him of a very famous baby who had started his life in a manger about two thousand years ago. Well, if you look at it in that light, my father admitted, maybe an underwear drawer wasn't such a bad deal.

The baby's name was also a direct consequence of the misunderstanding about its sexual identity. I've never been a fan of traditional family names and wanted to give my daughter a short and simple modern name. My father, though, yearned for a male descendant to carry on the Van der Vyver name and humbly asked me if the baby could possibly be named after him – if it was a boy, of course. I blithely answered yes, just to keep him happy.

Still, the moment the baby was lifted out of my body, I barely registered its sex. All I wanted to know was whether it was healthy and normal. Nothing else mattered. I vaguely remember hearing my mother gasp behind her surgical mask:

'*Maar hy het 'n tottermannetjie! Dis 'n seuntjie!*'[2] I stretched out my arms, already besotted with my son. Not even a split second of deception, confusion, puzzlement. Just pure joy. Probably the purest joy of my life.

Whenever I describe this birth, I have to fight my way through a jungle of clichés. My reactions and emotions; the behaviour of medical staff, family and friends; the profusion of flowers and visitors in my hospital room – the whole experience was so 'normal', so commonplace, so perfectly banal, compared to the silence and the loneliness of the previous birth. I learnt a valuable lesson, as a writer and as a human being. One can't always escape clichés and the commonplace. The banality of happiness is infinitely preferable to the particularity of despair.

And then I was foolish enough to think this was it. This was what I would be for the rest of my life: a single mother of a single child. Oh yes, and a writer, too. My first adult novel was published only a few weeks after Daniel's birth, and its success enabled me to buy a car, find a house and care for my child financially. So for me being a mother and being a writer will always remain intricately linked.

I forgot John Lennon's famous remark, 'Life is what happens while you're making other plans', until life happened to me in the form of a love affair with a Frenchman called Alain. I decided to move to France 'temporarily', just to give the relationship a go, and ended up having a child and promising to spend the rest of my life with him.

It was another unplanned pregnancy. Some of us never learn, do we? Alain and I discussed the issue of children like responsible adults and decided no, it wouldn't be a good idea. We already had three sons between the two of us, we really couldn't afford another child, and besides we were both getting rather long in the tooth. And then we went ahead, like irresponsible adolescents, and conceived another child.

This pregnancy produced a whole new set of fears, completely

---

2 'But he has a penis. It's a boy!'

different from my fears in previous pregnancies. At least I now knew it was possible for me to give birth to a healthy baby – but this time I was in a foreign country, far from my mother and all my female relatives and friends, and I had to speak a foreign language to doctors and medical staff. I soon learnt that when you don't speak their language well, medical staff tend to treat you like an idiot, overstating the obvious and not bothering to explain important procedures and possible consequences. Another new fear was linked to my age. Since I was on the wrong side of forty, the pregnancy was automatically regarded as high risk. I was about to become what doctors so unflatteringly call a 'geriatric' mother.

Yet, in spite of all my fears and phobias, both the old ones and the new ones, I gave birth – through another epidural Caesarean in a provincial French hospital – to another beautiful and healthy baby. The daughter that I'd expected the previous time had finally shown up. We decided to call her Mia, short and simple and modern, with the added advantage that her French father's and her Afrikaans mother's relatives would all be able to pronounce it in more or less the same way.

○

Back in my kitchen in a French village, I still haven't answered the question of particularity versus universality. I try to finish my cup of coffee calmly while the usual morning chaos erupts around me. By now everyone in the house is shouting at someone else. Daniel is shouting at me because he can't find any clean socks for school; Mia is shouting at Daniel, who has eaten the last of her favourite breakfast cereal; Alain is shouting at Daniel, who has left the bathroom floor all wet and slippery. Within moments I'm going to scream at the top of my lungs at all of them.

We're actually just another happy family, believe it or not. Happy in our *own* way.

Triptych

Sandra Dodson

I. Hell

It floated serenely in formaldehyde, eyes closed, looking strangely out of place among the other specimens on display in the science laboratory: a scorpion, a frog, a mouse. I flinched at seeing the scorpion's pincers so dangerously close to the foetus in the glass jar next to it, though I knew they were both dead. It was 1975. I was ten years old. We were at my older brother's school Open Day. I found it extraordinary that everyone – parents, aunts, uncles, cousins, brothers, sisters – should file so slowly, so quietly, past the baby, observing it as just another object of scientific interest. I wanted to know how it got there, whose it was, how it had died, why it was so pale, why it was in a jam jar. I asked my mother and father, but they looked embarrassed and said, '*Shh*, don't ask so many questions.'

Now, twenty-three years later, I have started a new job in the Exhibitions Department at the Museum of Modern Art in Oxford. A travelling exhibition titled *In Visible Light*, exploring photography's uneasy, shifting status between art and science, is scheduled to open in Stockholm on 20 November. I have travelled there to oversee the unpacking of the photographs from their crates and to advise the Swedish curator on the installation of the exhibition. Having never done anything like this before, I feel out of my depth. In fact, I'm still astonished that I've been given the job, as the interview had gone disastrously, I thought.

As I walk into the first gallery, white-walled, wooden-floored, church-like, I am overwhelmed by an image on the wall directly ahead of me, something not in the original list of works I had studied so thoroughly. It is a massively magnified, intricately detailed photograph of a foetus at ten weeks. It extends from just above the floor to almost ceiling height. I cannot look at it, but it is unavoidable – huge, almost grotesquely so, dwarfing all the other images. The curator walks over to me and remarks, 'Isn't it great?' I say, 'Yes, it's extraordinary.' 'I hope it's all right to augment the exhibition?' he asks. 'We have such big gallery spaces here.' I reply, 'Yes, yes, I'm sure it's fine. I'll check with MoMA.' Then I leave the room, overcome by nausea. Outside, in the frozen grounds of the museum, I retch.

Somehow the winter cold, the sterility of it, helps. Inside the museum building, the clinical environment of the room in which I am examining the photographs also offers a strange and unexpected relief. The conservators are dressed in white laboratory coats and talk softly in Swedish as they note signs of deterioration in some of the older photographs: fragile, valuable works by Eadweard Muybridge, Alphonse Bertillon and other nineteenth-century photographers, whose names are unfamiliar to me. They draw neat diagrams on crisp condition-checking forms. I am soothed by this orderliness, this sense of system, even as it draws attention to the dog-eared, haphazard state of the MoMA condition reports and the inadequacy of my own rough notes.

I find myself staring at a sequence of disturbing images documenting the artist's hospital treatment for breast cancer. I have read somewhere that the piece is intended as a critique of modern medicine's tendency to process individuals as biological specimens. I want to retch again. I pretend that I need to pee and am escorted by a female security guard to the toilet. We have to pass through several security gates to get there. Each is carefully unlocked and relocked. The woman waits for me outside the toilet, and I hope that she cannot hear me through the closed door.

○

Back in Oxford, the sky is monochrome. It is 25 November. Through the window of the hospital ward, I catch glimpses of birds swooping across the greyness. Situated in a low-lying building at the back of the hospital, the ward is far from the maternity section. I had struggled to find it at first. On arrival I fill in a form and am sent for a scan. I sit and wait alongside other pregnant women on the uncomfortable NHS chairs in the Radiography reception. The women talk animatedly with their husbands or boyfriends while they wait for the radiographer to call them in. I am alone. A sweet-faced girl, who can't be more than eighteen, with a tattoo across her flat belly and a pierced belly button, asks whether I'm enjoying the pregnancy, whether I'm going to find out if it's a boy or a girl. I say hesitantly, 'I'm not really sure what to expect,' then turn away. I feel like an impostor. The radiographer seems to detect it. She does not smile. She seems to be going through the motions. Afterwards I am sent to a counsellor. She asks how I felt when I saw the image of the foetus on the screen, the pulsating heart. I said I felt numb. She asks questions about the father, and I tell her that our relationship is breaking down. She says, 'You know, if you choose to go ahead, it's all right. Nobody here is judging you. We're just here to give support.'

On returning to the ward I undress and a nurse helps me into a white cotton gown. Then I lie on the bed and wait. There are five other beds in the ward, occupied mostly by young girls, visibly anxious. Some have boyfriends at their sides. A fair-haired girl opposite is alone, weeping quietly. Nobody seems as old as I am. Then the cubicle curtains are drawn and a doctor comes to my bedside. She is South African. I know it from her face and manner even before she speaks. I hate this enforced intimacy, this complicity, as much as she does, and I sense her discomfort as she describes the procedure. She averts her eyes. A nurse wheels me into the operating theatre. I avoid looking at the tray of instruments. The anaesthetist says, 'OK, just relax, here we go.' As I feel consciousness slipping away, I think of the way the tall summer grass moves in the wind on the hillside opposite my family home in KwaZulu-Natal. After the operation, I find myself asking repeatedly, 'How big was the foetus, how big was the foetus?' Nobody will answer me. Nobody seems to tell me anything.

My boyfriend fetches me the same day. We do not speak.

We know the relationship is over. We return to our basement flat, which smells of damp. The musty odour had nauseated me for ten weeks and, though the sick sensation has now gone, I still find the smell intolerable. I am bleeding so heavily I think I am dying. The first time I shower, I am shocked to find milk trickling absurdly from my breasts. At first I do not know what it is. Then I understand. And I sit down in the shower and weep. I have aborted a foetus, and my body will not believe it, is biologically programmed not to. It believes it has given birth to a ten-week-old baby and must sustain it. For three weeks I am so depressed I cannot leave the house. I phone the museum and tell them that I have had an operation to remove a uterine cyst, and have reacted badly to the anaesthetic. The landlady comes to fetch the rent. She tells me, in passing, that she and her husband, a choirmaster at one of the colleges, are opening a refuge for unmarried pregnant girls. Being committed Catholics, she explains, they are wholly opposed to abortion.

II. Purgatory

It is early autumn, almost a year later. I have moved to a house in South Oxford, across the river. It has been recently renovated. I like the restored wooden floors and sash windows, the smell of fresh paint. My housemates are lovely. Cait especially, with her outrageous laugh. But today, a Saturday, I am on my own. Cait and Giles are away for the weekend. I am lonely. The house feels cold, empty, as if the spaces between things have inexplicably increased. Physical objects seem suddenly estranged, contained, separate. Even the walls have retreated. I sit at the dining-room table, in a pool of weak sunlight, writing a letter to a friend in South Africa. I am trying to find a way of telling him what has happened since we last corresponded, but I cannot find the words. I am unsure whether I want to tell *him* specifically, or whether I simply have a need to write about it. Either way, the pen feels useless in my hand.

There is a knock at the door. I get up, eagerly, to answer it, and am half disappointed, half intrigued, to find a gypsy woman standing outside. In her hand is a worn Sainsbury's shopping bag. She has the Romany chestnut complexion, dark eyes, and thick dark hair beneath a colourful headscarf. Over layered, mismatched clothing, she wears an old cardigan. Some of the buttons are missing. Looking at her, I remember the beautiful gypsy outfit my mother made for my dress-up box when I was a child.

She takes a pile of white lace doilies from the Sainsbury's bag, and asks if I would like to buy some. Only ten pounds for five. I tell her that I do not use doilies, though I admit that the handwork is beautiful, intricate. She says that she will tell my fortune for free if I buy one. I have never had faith in fortune-tellers, but something makes me agree to this. I invite her inside. She sits opposite me at the dining-room table and takes my hand. It is a long time since anyone has held my hand, and I am comforted by her touch.

She tells me in a strangely disturbing monotone that I am lonely. She tells me that I am respected at work. She tells me that I will go on to have three children and that they will always live near to me. She says other things, more or less plausible, which I can no longer remember. Then she looks directly into my eyes and tells me that I have done something for which I feel deeply guilty.

I know on one level that she has probably said something similar to everyone else who has allowed her this sort of intimacy. But on another level, I believe that she *knows*. She tells me that I must trust her. That if I do not trust, I will suffer under some kind of curse for ten years. Then she asks for all the money I have in the house. She asks me to trust that she will bring it back. By now I know that she is manipulating me, and that she has no intention of returning. But I also know that I cannot refuse. I have only a few pounds in my wallet. The amount seems inadequate. So I cycle to the nearest Barclays Bank cash-point and take out three hundred pounds. There is nothing left in my account. I give the money to her in a sealed envelope and she leaves.

A few weeks later I hear that my former landlady has developed Alzheimer's. She walks familiar streets and cannot find her way home.

III. Paradise

One night, in November 2002, I dream of light. It is the amber light found on the Cape coast towards evening, in the fullness of summer. There is little other detail in the dream. The next day I find myself missing – with unusual intensity – a friend I have known from childhood. His name is Andrew. He returned to South Africa in 1999 after nearly a decade in London. I look up his telephone number. We haven't spoken for months and he sounds surprised, happy, to hear from me. We talk for an hour or more, sensing one another's reluctance to hang up. I'm about to put down the receiver when he says, out of the blue, 'Why don't you come home?' I feel the word before I hear it. With the force of desire, it rushes through me, a sensation at the same time deeply familiar and overwhelming, like something experienced for the first time. For a moment I cannot speak. But I know the answer. I want, more than anything, to come home.

In September 2003, a few days before my birthday, I return. Andrew is with me. We travel to my parents' thatched fishing cottage on the Lions River, in the KwaZulu-Natal Midlands. This is where I spent many childhood holidays, and where my father himself spent much of his childhood and early adult life. While a student, he would take friends there to fish and swim on weekends. There is a visitors' book, dating back to the fifties, which records everything from the size of rainbow trout caught in the river, to levels of summer rainfall, to the naming of the various fishing and swimming spots: 'Otters Pool', 'Lady Barbara's Bath', 'Madoda's Reach', 'Long Pool'.

Forty-eight years previously, almost to the day, the visitors' book records the twenty-first birthday party of a friend of my father's. It contains the signatures of all who were there, including my mother, then an eighteen-year-old girl in her second year at university. She had gone reluctantly, having been persuaded by a friend that she needed a break from swotting for exams. And so it happened that she met my father, then aged nineteen. By all accounts it was love at first sight, though my mother likes to pretend otherwise. In the years that follow, the visitors' book records their marriage; our births and christenings, some at the local church; our heights and weights; our early drawing and writing attempts; our school prizes. Later it records my siblings' respective marriages, and the births and christenings of my niece and nephews.

It is spring and the massed azaleas are in full flower. I rest on the bed and listen to the familiar sound of the river down in the valley, the high-pitched humming of the Christmas beetles and the *tick tick* of the old geyser. Then I hear thunder and the soft, soporific sound of rain on the thatch. I realise that I have not spent a night in the cottage since childhood. While visiting from England as an adult, I had always stayed in my parents' house next door, the cottage being reserved for guests with families.

Andrew and I are now expecting our first child.

The next day I phone a private midwife in Pietermaritzburg. I tell her that I plan to give birth in hospital, but would like a midwife rather than an obstetrician to deliver our baby. We meet in simply furnished consulting rooms adjoining her home. She is a friendly woman in her mid-forties, with a reassuringly practical, down-to-earth manner. I like her at once. I trust her. The walls are brightly decorated with photographs of the babies she has delivered, many of them water births, attended at home. Water birth, she explains, is the least traumatic way for a baby to adjust to life outside the cushioned, amniotic environment of the womb. When she asks if I would consider giving birth at home, I say that I will keep an open mind, but I am concerned about possible complications. Her preference is obvious, but she makes no attempt to persuade me. Instead, she tells me that the experience of labour and birth is profoundly influenced by a woman's state of mind. The crucial thing is to feel comfortable, safe, supported, wherever you are.

The days pass. We swim in the river and walk in the indigenous bush, where the air is cool. Everything seems to happen slowly, with my belly by now low and heavy. A week or so before my due date, we see three young otters cavorting in the reeds, their coats black and shiny wet.

Now it is the following week, around eleven p.m. on 4 November 2003. Lying awake next to Andrew, I can just make out the dark shape of the rafters above the bed, the steep pitch of the thatched roof. There is a dull ache in my lower back, and I am struggling to sleep. Then suddenly, around midnight, I feel it: a slow, deep-down clamping, tightening, twisting, and gradual release. The feeling comes again, more intensely, about fifteen minutes later. I wake Andrew and, sleepily, he begins to time the duration between each spasm. At seven a.m. we phone the midwife. She tells me to go for a walk, to keep moving. And so we walk together down the hill to the river, along the bank, downstream, then back up the hill past the ruin of the old caretaker's dwelling and the overgrown vegetable garden. We see a solitary fish eagle at the top of a pine tree, surveying the water below. Every ten minutes or so I feel the grip of another contraction and bend over, close to the ground. I try to concentrate on my breathing, remembering how, as a child, I used to do yoga exercises with my mother, breathing deeply in and out. I remember the diagrams of the female reproductive organs on the pink exercise charts.

The midwife arrives at ten a.m. I am relieved to see her. She examines me and says reassuringly, 'If you'd like to go to hospital, I think we should leave now. If you'd feel more comfortable staying here, that's fine. I have everything I need for a home birth.' Her matter-of-fact tone surprises me, as if I expect something out of the ordinary, an impending crisis of some kind, deserving a more urgent response. There is no hint of anxiety in her voice. I consider her question, carefully. Outside it has begun to rain, and mist has obscured the hillside opposite the cottage. I imagine possible delays as we travel along muddy farm roads and through misty stretches on the motorway. I anticipate the discomfort of the car journey and the clinical environment of the hospital, where Andrew cannot stay with me overnight. Then I think of staying in this familiar place, in the care of a woman whose professional judgement I trust, with my loved ones close by. I decide to stay.

At around five p.m., Andrew runs a bath for me in the deep enamel tub where, aged thirteen, I'd first experienced a period, the sight of blood in the water arousing both shock and excitement. Kneeling in the water, I imagine my cervix opening slowly, slowly, while the baby moves ever downwards, pushed by the contracting uterus, turning sideways as it passes through the pelvis, knowing instinctively what to do.

Suddenly an agonising weight presses into my groin. I start to bellow and Andrew, caught equally off guard, lurches to his feet to call the midwife, who is setting up her equipment in the bedroom next door.

From then on I am both present and not present. The pain obliterates me. I see and hear the midwife from a vast distance. At times I feel as if I am being dragged out to sea by some treacherous undertow while Andrew tries to hold me back. In the stainless steel of the tap I see my face, distorted, unrecognisable. I seem to recall the midwife pulling on her gloves and asking me to stand up so that she and Andrew can lift me out of the bath. I remember the effort of trying, and my failure, finding my legs too weak, the pressure in my pelvis too severe. A soft voice says something about delivering my baby in the water. I remember the words, 'Just relax.' Then I am aware of someone handling me gently, laying me back in the warmth, while the same familiar voice asks me to push. I breathe deeply and bear down, though I barely have the strength. Then, when I feel close to drowning, the voice reassures me that the head is crowning: I must take rapid, shallow breaths, and soon it will be over. An impossible sensation of stretching, stretching, and now someone takes my hand and guides it to where I feel something hard, expecting to find softness. The top of the baby's head, with its waxy coating of vernix, pushes against my hand. I start to cry. Then, with an involuntary push, the head is out, supported under the water, and I must bear down once more to release the limbs and body. Suddenly, the midwife lifts our daughter out and into my arms. She is pink as a sea lily, her little form already unfurling, her feet and hands wrinkled from the brine. Held in the curve of my arm, she nuzzles my wet breasts, smelling the sweetness of milk. It is 5:45 p.m.

Andrew walks through the rain to tell my parents that they have a granddaughter: Beatrice, meaning 'bringer of joy'. They arrive at the cottage with supper on a tray and a bottle of red wine. Beatrice is already sleeping, warmly swaddled. We light a fire in the fireplace.

Outside the mist has lifted. Looking out of the window, into the dusk, I see the tall grass rippling on the hillside across the river.

A Love Triangle

Ronel Herrendoerfer & Anneke Kamfer-Sloman

It started as an adventure. I was on my way home with a friend when we decided to get a video. As we walked into the Rondebosch video store, I saw an advertisement stuck in the window.

Surrogate mother needed

Couple looking for a loving woman to carry their baby.
Genetically, the baby will be completely theirs.
We are looking for someone who fits the following description:

Must have at least one child of her own
Non-smoker and non-drinker
Preferably between 23 and 35 years old
Must have a history of uncomplicated pregnancy
Must have support of family and friends
Must not be afraid of doctors
Must be prepared to have an HIV test
Must be in good health and live healthily.

My friend went inside, but I couldn't stop reading. Before we left I took down the telephone number.

When I got back to Grassy Park, I told my sister that I was thinking of becoming a surrogate mother. She looked at me like I was crazy and said, 'Why would you want to do something like *that*?' But I phoned the number anyway. Nobody answered, so I left a message and waited. I remember thinking, *It will never happen*. It was such a long shot. But then the lady phoned me back. Her name was Anneke.

130

When I met her I liked her straight away. She was very warm and friendly. She said she had been trying to have children for years and now she was approaching forty. So it had been a long time. She had done IVF three times, but it hadn't worked. She'd also had operations to have her fibroids removed. This was her last chance. I could see how badly she wanted a child. I knew then that I wanted to carry a baby for her. But I really didn't think she would go for me.

Later she told me that I was the third caller to answer the advert, but as soon as she had talked to me, she knew I was the person she was looking for. It felt right. She said she liked me from the start. She liked that I was down to earth and straightforward.

We didn't talk about money. She just told me what the problem was and asked me why I wanted to be a surrogate. She also asked me questions about my family. I told her surrogacy was something I had wanted to do for a long time, but I thought it only happened on TV. I didn't think it was possible here in South Africa. I couldn't believe that I had found someone wanting me to be a surrogate for her.

Then I told her about my family. About my daughter, who was eleven at that time, and about my late sister's two children, who also live with us. (My older sister died of a heart attack in 2001). I explained that I fell pregnant when I was in standard 9 and went back to school the following year to do my matric. My mother worked, but a lady down the road watched my baby for me. It was difficult, but not that bad. I got through my matric even though I didn't think I would make it.

I told Anneke that because I already had a family, I didn't want another baby of my own. I couldn't afford it, not as a single working mother who wanted to be able to give her children what they needed. My life was stressful enough without a baby. I didn't want us to struggle. No, I definitely didn't want another child of my own. But I would do it for someone else, especially someone who wanted a baby so much. To do it for her would be nice. I love being pregnant; it isn't difficult for me.

There was another reason I wanted to be a surrogate.

Something I don't think I told Anneke then. When I was very young, my cousin would fall pregnant and then lose the baby. It happened again and again. She couldn't carry a child. I saw how sad it made her, and that feeling stayed with me as I grew up. I remember thinking then that somebody should just do it for her. I would have done it. But I was too young, I couldn't. That feeling was always with me. Now at last I could do something about it.

At the end of our meeting we agreed that we all needed to think about it. After a week we would meet again. But before the week was up, Anneke and her husband phoned me. It was a Sunday and they were driving home after a weekend in the Karoo. She wanted to know what I had decided and I told her I had made up my mind. If she wanted to go for it, I was there. I could hear her shouting with excitement. It was so nice.

○

From day one I told my daughter and my nieces: 'I'm going to have someone's baby for her. This aunty also loves babies, but she can't have one on her own. I'm going to have one for her. So that she can love it a lot, like Mommy loves you.' They understood. In fact my daughter has often said, 'Mommy, I want to do what you have done.' I tell her, 'OK, maybe when you're an adult. But you must have your own family first.'

Before we could go for IVF, I had to be screened by a psychologist. The decision rested with her alone. It was so scary. She asked me how I coped with my daughter and my sister's children, and how they would feel about me being a surrogate. She asked me about relationships, and I told her that I had had the same boyfriend for eight years.

I tried to be as calm as I could be in the interview. I knew I couldn't blow it! I told her that I was a tranquil, easygoing person, which is true. But I didn't tell her about the bigger picture: *Don't push me too far, I can get huffy!* I also told her that I am a person who looks at a situation very closely before I do anything about it.

132

I was so happy and relieved when the psychologist gave the go-ahead and we could arrange to have our first IVF treatment.

We went to see the professor who would do the IVF. I didn't really like him, not at first. He was like someone from the old South Africa. But I accepted that he was the expert and that Anneke needed him.

When the first implant didn't work, I think I felt even worse than Anneke did, and I know she was really sad. I felt so bad for her because I knew she really wanted it to work. I felt I'd failed her, especially since we were so sure about ourselves. But we tried again.

After the second time, my back was sore for a week and I thought something was wrong. I phoned Anneke and we went to the doctor together and he did a pregnancy test. I was at work, at Sweets from Heaven in Canal Walk, when I heard the result. 'Are you sitting down?' Anneke asked. Then she shouted, 'We're pregnant!' I remember saying, 'Calm down, calm down,' but of course she couldn't be calm. The pain I had felt had been a good pain. I told her, 'You see, good things do happen.' There was even more good news waiting around the corner. When we went for the first scan, we discovered it wasn't just one baby, it was twins!

It was very nice being pregnant with someone else's babies. The only downside was that I got terrible morning sickness. That was a real strain, because I had to continue working until just before the birth, getting up early and coming home at about six thirty or seven. I used to commute by bus all the way from Grassy Park to Canal Walk and back again. The people at work didn't know I was pregnant. I never told them.

I thought the nausea would get better after the first three months, but it didn't. I used to dread brushing my teeth in the morning. The minute I did, I'd be sick. And of course, nobody was sympathetic. Now that I was pregnant, I couldn't complain, because it was something I had chosen to do. My sister wasn't happy with me and it put a strain on my other relationships too. My boyfriend wasn't so keen at first, but he came around. My sister also came around in her own way. When I got home tired from work one day, she said, 'I'll cook for you. It's fine.'

I knew that if my mother had been alive she would probably have killed me. I probably wouldn't have done it. But now things were different. I felt strong. When people said, 'Are you mad? Why are you doing this?' I would say, 'Because I like it.' Simple.

My mom's sister wasn't very happy. But I always used to say to her, 'You've got children. I've got children. It's nice to have children. This lady can't have children. I want to make her happy.' When Anneke met my aunty, and my aunty liked her, she also came to understand why I was doing this, and became more involved. She'd bring a chair for me to put my feet up, kind things like that.

I remember Anneke saying she didn't know how I coped when my family or friends weren't supportive. She was always very sympathetic. I knew that if something *did* go wrong, and I got depressed, Anneke would understand. She would know where that feeling came from.

Anneke was great throughout the pregnancy. I know it must have been difficult for her. She told me that people would ask her how she was coping, knowing that her babies were growing inside someone else. They wanted to know if she was afraid that I would change my mind and want to keep the babies. But she never doubted me. We trusted each other.

She would phone me every day to check how I was. If she was in town and saw something good for pregnant mothers to eat, she would buy it for me. She made sure I ate healthily. I even managed to give up coffee, and I *love* coffee. I don't know how I did it, but I did.

Sometimes we'd go shopping together for maternity clothes. She'd phone me and say, 'I saw this lovely maternity dress . . . If you don't like it, we can take it back.' When people saw us in the maternity section, and asked how many months pregnant I was, I would always say, '*We* are so many months. How do *we* look?'

We became really close. It was *our* pregnancy. Anneke once told me that she was experiencing what lots of men must feel when their wives are pregnant. They are so involved, but it's not them carrying the baby. When we had the scans it helped her to feel more connected.

I remember calling her the first time the babies kicked. She came over to my house in Grassy Park right away. 'I'll make them kick for you,' I told her. Then I patted my tummy and said, 'Come, babies, kick for your mum,' and they kicked. Whatever happened with them, I would tell her.

When I was a month pregnant we had a scare. I started bleeding. The pain was so bad. I thought, *Not this!* I phoned Anneke. We didn't know what to expect when I had the scan, but both the babies were still there. Anneke just started crying. I got off work for a while and she took me to Gordon's Bay for a holiday with my family, so that I could have a rest.

○

People often ask me if it was hard to give the babies up. They think I must have bonded with them. But it wasn't hard, because I didn't let myself bond. Psychologically I shut myself off. I would say to myself, *These are not mine.* I wouldn't dream about them or think what they looked like. At times, when they kicked too much, I'd say, 'Come on, don't do that.' Sometimes I'd play music to them or talk to them. But I never bonded.

In the eighth month of our pregnancy, Anneke and her husband went to a wedding in Sweden. Her husband was going to be best man. Things had been going well, and we weren't worried. They had discussed the trip with me and I encouraged them to go. Anneke and I even got in one last bit of maternity shopping.

In the week before they left, we went for a final scan. Everything was fine. But while they were gone my blood pressure went sky-high. Her husband's parents, who were helping me, took me to the doctor. Anneke's mother-in-law was very worried.

The doctor told me I had pre-eclampsia. It was odd, because I didn't feel anything with it. I felt fine. But I had to stay in hospital. What really depressed me was that it was Fathers' Day and I wanted to be home with my boyfriend and my kids. I complained to the doctor. It was only after he told me that he also wanted to be at home, and that it was because of me that he was in the hospital, that I came to my senses.

I was so relieved that they made it back for the birth. They *had* to be there after all we had been through. Anneke told me when she saw me how worried she had been. I don't think she could relax on that holiday. I spoke to Anneke's father for the first time the night before the Caesar. I had only spoken to him on the phone before. He said, 'It's so nice what you're doing for my daughter.' That meant a lot to me.

When Anneke and her husband walked into the operating theatre, the nurses looked surprised and asked them who they were. They shouted proudly, 'We are the parents!' The gynae joked, saying, 'Tickets, please!' Anneke and her husband sat down near me, as close as they could be without getting in the way. My fiancé held my hand all the time.

Having a Caesar was strange. I had had a natural birth with my daughter. The first twin took a long time to come out. There was a problem because she had swallowed some fluid and had to be given oxygen. While she was being helped, the next one popped óut. They were so tiny.

The doctors said they were proud of me. Even the professor I hadn't liked congratulated me. He came up to me and said, 'You did great. The babies are great. You are a remarkable lady.' It felt good that he had had a change of heart.

It was lovely to have everyone fussing over me. I felt like a queen. The doctors and nurses would come up to me and tell me I did so well! They had given me something to dry up the breast milk, so I wasn't uncomfortable. It dried up immediately. There was no sensation, nothing.

The twins had to stay in post-natal intensive care for two weeks before they could go home. But I was able to leave hospital after a few days. Everyone was worried about me going home after the birth. We had agreed that we wouldn't make contact during the first three months. But after the first week Anneke phoned me. She was more worried about me than about herself. She asked if I was miserable. I said, 'Am I supposed to be?' Then I reassured her that I was fine. I told her I felt good about what I had done. I asked her, 'How are you?' I knew it was tough for her. She had two babies to look after suddenly.

She wanted to breast-feed, feeling it would be good for bonding, but the doctors didn't want to give her drugs to stimulate milk. They said it wouldn't be good for her or the babies. That was hard for her.

After a month I saw them again. Anneke looked worn out. I asked her, 'What's happening?' She said, 'I'm adjusting.' I recall she was struggling to change one of the twin's nappies. She'd put the nappy under the baby, but lifted the baby's legs up too high. It was difficult to watch her trying over and over. I was itching to change the nappy for her, but I didn't take over. I just suggested what she might do differently. I think she appreciated it.

After that we would phone each other and chat.

When the babies were three months old, I went to Anneke's house with my daughter and nieces. It was the first time my children had seen the twins. Anneke gave one of the twins to me to feed. I had her on my arm. It was funny to think that this little stranger had once been inside me.

Three years after the twins were born, I became a surrogate again and had a baby boy for a couple who couldn't have a second child. I wanted to have a natural birth, but the parents weren't comfortable with it, so I had another Caesar. Unfortunately, I got an abscess afterwards and was in intensive care for a long time. Now I have a scar all the way down my stomach. That makes me a bit upset, but I would do it again. My doctor doesn't want me to. But I'm only thirty-four and I'm ready.

Anneke is still good to me. She always remembers my birthday and we go out. The babies are now five years old. One looks just like her father, but she has the character of her mother. The other looks just like her mother, but she has the character of her father. I am so proud of them.

○

Postscript

How can I describe the moments when, looking across the gleaming expanse of the theatre floor and past the glittering instruments, I first laid eyes on the minute, bloodied forms of my babies? I can't. Suffice it to say that I saw it all through a veil of tears, with unintelligible sounds welling up from somewhere deep inside. Photographs show me with my hands clasped to my mouth, red eyes wide in disbelief, my body bent forward as if I'm about to take off at speed. The theatre cap had slipped down and was almost over my eyes. All in all, I looked like the village idiot, but I was oblivious. This was the moment.

Even though I couldn't hold my babies on that first day, I felt an intense bond between us from the moment I saw them. There was nothing strange, distant or 'other' about them. They were familiar to me, in the fullest sense of the word.

We left the ICU late that night, but the drive home felt wrong. Close friends came over to celebrate with champagne, but even as I was smiling and talking, relating the momentous events of the day, I felt edgy and displaced. It didn't feel right to be at home, with those two small parts of me nowhere in evidence. Gradually, over the two weeks they spent in the ICU, that sense of unreality when I was not with them diminished.

The ICU staff believed strongly in 'kangaroo care'. When the twins' condition had stabilised and they had shed some of the tubes that confined them to the incubator, my husband and I were allowed to spend as many hours as we wished holding one or both of them as close as possible. Feeling those small, warm bodies on my skin was like nothing I had ever felt before. Every cell in my body seemed to plump up with love.

Ronel would come to the ICU regularly to see the girls and was allowed to hold them. The nurses fussed over her, making her feel special and appreciated. She was discharged after three days. I went with her when she had her stitches out and she paid one more visit to the twins before they were discharged. Then we did not see each other for about a month. I spoke to her on the phone regularly and repeated our offer of paying for counselling if she felt the need, but she wouldn't take it up.

She said that she never felt regret or sadness, only a very deep sense of satisfaction, of knowing that she had done 'something good'.

Ronel's gift of twins has given me something I thought I would never have: a family of my own. How I love to see their shiny little heads bowed together over one book!

My cup runneth over.

Invisible

Willemien de Villiers

Reluctant to return to the landscape of birth, I continue to avoid writing the story I need to write. It is possible that my resistance is influenced by research: I am currently immersed in the infamous Boer War Battle of Spionkop. My personal birth narrative seems similarly stuck on some distant battlefield where abandoned fragments of memory lie buried in shallow trenches.

So I decide to plant spring bulbs instead and wait for the story to find me. I carry five shallow clay pots to a sunny corner of my garden and start filling them with dark, crumbling soil. The bulbs are indigenous – *Amaryllis belladonna* and yellow Ifafa lilies.

Whenever I garden, I have silent conversations with my father, and it is to him that I confess that I don't want to write about my grandmother Kate, who was born on the day that her three-year-old sister was buried, and whose middle name, Maria, was changed to Mara, a bitter, biblical *memento mori*.

I don't want to write about my mother's birth, which preceded the death of her grandfather by twelve hours. The bitter second name was swiftly passed on, this time as my mother's first name.

I don't want to write about my own birth either, after which I lay swaddled and separated from my mother for three days while doctors fought to stem the bleeding that threatened to drain her life away. Life and death, inextricably linked all the way down my maternal line.

I never managed to ask my father whether he held me, and nursed me, during those long hours. Nervous of the need such a question would reveal, I hesitate to ask it even now, so many years after his death.

As I lift the first swollen globe into its prepared hole, a

fragment appears in my mind. Some fusion of fact and fiction. I water the planted bulbs and walk inside to wash my hands. Sitting down in front of my computer, I open a new document and start to type.

During the seventh month of Inge's pregnancy, the tall display cabinet that used to stand in her parents' lounge starts appearing in her dreams. In these dreams, Inge – who seems to be the only solid object amidst several floating, translucent layers – opens the doors of the cabinet and removes her mother's treasures one by one, offering them to her father's reflection.

My parents never owned such a display cabinet, but my grandmother did, filled with books and a few ugly porcelain statues of little shepherd boys and girls. Cheap figurines cast from overused moulds, their faces, underneath milky layers of underfired glaze, seemed rubbed out. An ever-present spectre during my childhood visits there, the glassy surface of the cabinet's tall, closed doors reflected the room in which it stood, the entrance hall of my grandparents' house beyond, as well as their bedroom, with its ornately carved, hinged wooden screen, hiding their plump, wide bed. It was here that my father sometimes took afternoon naps after Sunday lunch visits.

For my story, I want to place my grandmother on that plump bed, giving birth to her three daughters and two stillborn sons, but I can't, because that was not how it happened – she gave birth to my mother inside a provincial hospital in Kroonstad.

Her father is lying on her mother's side of the plump, wide bed, the reflected curve of his back as flimsy as the peel-off stickers Inge used to collect and swap as a child with her friends. Although her father lost his eyesight in a hunting accident at the age of eight – shooting springbok on a farm near Noupoort in the Karoo – inside Inge's dreams he can always see.

A black cloth, embroidered with mythical six-legged animals, hangs on the inside back panel of Inge's mother's cabinet. It forms the backdrop to her collection of treasures: two green glass vases with frosted handles and sturdy feet (decorated with ornate, curled-up fern leaves that remind Inge of green embryos); an old framed etching of a melancholy woman with a rust-coloured plait resting heavily across one breast; four glazed clay horses; three multicoloured beaded balls; rows of books; an untidy, well-thumbed stack of tarot cards tumbling its many mysteries onto the bottom shelf; a multitude of grey-and-black striped stones.

'Just look at that!' her father exclaims as he turns Inge's offering to the light. 'Isn't it beautiful?'

My fingers hover above the keyboard. My father had twenty-twenty vision until the day he died, curled on his side in a hospital bed in Bloemfontein. He fell ill while building a rockery in my brother's garden, now filled with dusky green succulents. My father loved the rocks and stones, the red earth and white thorns of our country's northern landscape. Although he had the eyesight of an eagle, I have felt hidden from him all my life.

When Inge wakes up, the taste of the dream lingers, similar to the peppery bite of nasturtium. Growing up, Inge was intrigued by the fact that her father was unable to see her, and, by way of testing her invisibility, would sometimes confront his calm, smiling face by sticking out her tongue and rolling her eyes.

So that her father could choose which colours to wear, Inge's mother sewed discreetly placed buttons onto each article of clothing he owned: one button for blue (the colour of a warm, sunny day); two for red (blood flowing from an awkwardly bent antelope neck, biltong sliced with a blood-streaked knife, his mother's fragrant lips); three for green (first shoots on the umbrella thorn); four for white (the smooth enamel of his childhood bath, painted lines on the main road to town, clouds); five small buttons for yellow and orange (warm mealies, dripping with melted butter, flowering aloes).

No buttons for black or brown.

Inge's father never wore purple.

On rainy days, young Inge would sit on the carpet of their lounge, pulling objects from a bag for her father to feel and examine. The bag of black was filled with stones, jet beads, black feathers, a black electrical cord, a hairdryer, two round picture frames, a mug, a comb, a black lock of her hair. Looking at their refection in the panelled doors of the display cabinet, she would press the soft pad of his thumb over the hole in the centre of an old LP record from his mother's collection, and scratch his nails across its liquorice grooves.

'I still remember,' he would say then, balancing the vinyl disk on his palm. 'All this music . . . and it weighs almost nothing.'

I get up from behind my desk and remove a slim, orange-spined volume from my bookshelf: my twenty-two-year-old copy of Janet Balaskas's *Active Birth*. Opening it randomly, I find the familiar grainy black-and-white photograph of a woman with nipples the size and colour of small terracotta saucers. Leaning against her husband, who is wearing an inexplicable smile along with his white surgeon's cap, the photographed woman's posture suggests complete surrender. A bearded man crouches at her feet, peering up between her legs. Her eyes are closed, her breath caught between her lips. Another photograph shows her newborn baby suckling at one of her ample breasts. A pale grey umbilical cord dangles between her fingers, not yet cut. She is laughing open-mouthed, triumphant, looking straight at me.

Ten days before the birth, Inge walks aimlessly through a large shopping centre, pausing in front of a display in the window of a toy shop: battery-operated, life-size cats lie curled up in soft baskets, their fake-fur bellies inflating and deflating as if breathing. She is reminded of her father's reassuring murmur as he stroked their Siamese cat while she gave birth to the first of a litter of four kittens.

Armed with a brand-new vocabulary, Inge feels well prepared for the imminent birth – *oedema, perineum, anterior lip, pelvic inlet, pubic arch, episiotomy, pethidine, Braxton-Hicks, Lamaze, kneeling position, half-kneeling, half-squatting, transition* – and that night she dreams of finding small, lifelike dolls in each of the rooms of her house. Their plastic eyes stare past her as she rests her

143

fingertips against their cold rubber chests, rising and falling, rising and falling.

Waking up, Inge notices three gulls circling high above her lawn. Dark chocolate butterflies are skimming blades of buffalo grass, sipping at the dew collected there.

The distant sea is as loud as a train rushing past.

Seven nights before the birth of my first child, I fell asleep in front of my grandmother's tall display cabinet. I inherited it after her death, and had by then filled it with my own treasures – two burnished Venda pots, seven small discs woven from colourful telephone wire, and one of my sculptures: stacked ceramic soup bowls placed on a plinth of fused, glazed cutlery. Newspaper reports of murder and domestic mayhem are engraved on the outside surface of the bowls. A single spoon, resting inside the top bowl, overflows with word-embossed bisqued shards.

Curled up in front of the cabinet, I dreamt I was waiting for my father at an unfamiliar station. I noticed rows of faces peering through the narrow, oblong windows of a stationary train, featureless balloons tied to the chrome frames of the oxblood fake-leather seats.

'I have to talk to you about the statistical improbability of love,' my father said, suddenly appearing at the open door of the train, holding on to my shoulder as he jumped from the metal step to the grubby platform.

'I'm going to have a baby,' I told him as he steered my heavy body deftly through the milling crowds.

'So I see,' he replied.

The dream shifted to the familiar bus journey I used to make to visit Celeste, my childhood friend (a girl my mother despised). I chose always to sit far away from the spitting-mad driver and his hurled insults.

'You're such a nuisance,' the bus driver hissed into my sleeping ears as I got out of the bus and walked with my father in tow past the Catholic boarding school, where nuns roosted like giant birds of prey and an anorexic Jesuswoman hung from a copper cross against a bone-china cup of sky. Birds stuck to its sides like tea leaves.

'Look!' I exclaimed, and my father nodded his head.

Only an hour's drive separated us, yet my father and I seldom talked. Maybe that explains why he took up residence in my dreams, an omniscient narrator whispering footnotes.

During the last five days of her pregnancy, Inge continues to make delicate botanical sketches: of arum skin so velvet-smooth she finds herself licking at the thick, absorbent watercolour paper, and of a recently discovered stag-horn fern growing against the trunk of a ficus in her garden.

'Green, but not dark like your pants,' she says out loud, rubbing at the kicking heel of her restless baby. 'More grey, as if mixed with the chest feathers of a pigeon.'

She sees her father, wearing a shirt of soft corduroy with five hidden buttons, lightly pressing his fingertips against the spiky leaves of a potted aloe before picking a single, small orange bell from the flaming raceme.

In the manner of a love-struck teenager, Inge scribbles different names in the margins of her paintings, practising, practising: *Mia, Hannah, Leah, Thérèsa, Petra, Malika.* Every now and then a boy's name manages to gallop in: *Markus, Thomas, David, Aram,* as well as her father's name, *Leon.*

While searching for a name, Inge tilts her head, listening, and hears her mother's voice. Her mother, who phones daily from her telephone next to her plump, wide bed, still hidden behind the carved wooden screen.

Nearly three months have passed. Several glossy green shoots now push through the soil in the pots outside, and while watering them, I am once more talking to my father. An unplanned telling of my first labour pains, of my first daughter's reluctance to leave the safety of my womb, and of my second daughter's unseemly haste to exit that hand-me-down space previously occupied by her sister.

Before sitting down at my computer to finish Inge's story, I fetch my father's blue-framed photograph from my bookshelf and place it next to me on my desk. His head is slightly tilted to the left, half hidden in shadow. For the first time, I see that I have inherited his hesitant, close-lipped smile.

I love you, I think, and notice that his eyes look straight into mine.

When Inge arrives at the hospital, she walks slowly to the natural childbirth ward, leaning against her husband. Crawling to the pile of cushions in the corner of the birthing room, she grunts at the smiling midwife walking past. Down the corridor, past the green bathroom and the white kitchen, she can hear the sound of clanging stainless steel.

'A parallelogram of pain,' her father says, squatting down next to her. 'You must lean into it.'

Inge floats in a warm tub of water, then walks up and down the gleaming corridor. Her husband shuffles awkwardly at her side. Elated, her baby kicks and kicks until the warm liquid streams from between her mother's legs. 'Let go of me!' Inge screams, and her husband jumps back.

Her hair is sweat-plastered to her cheeks, her eyes unfocused; a convicted criminal already serving time. Between contractions, she glimpses the soul of her child.

When Inge is finally ready to surrender her baby, she notices her father in a shadowed corner of the room. He is holding out a pot of yellow lilies in full bloom.

'Look,' he says, as Inge's husband lifts their daughter onto her soft belly. 'Isn't it beautiful?'

The Postcard

Reviva Schermbrucker

I absent-mindedly scan the postcard from Linda, childless in Amsterdam, then flip it over.

Mid-conversation with Sally, I suck in my breath. 'Yikes!'

'What?'

'I'm staring at . . . at, um . . . a birth,' I say into the phone, bringing the image out of the telephone-nook gloom.

The figure is – or should it be figures are? – in green speckled stone, slicked in high gloss. The mother is squatting, her full weight balanced dramatically on the tips of her stony toes. The big head juts out, eyes blank, mouth open with its row of cartoon-perfect teeth and lips drawn back in a near-mechanical grimace. Collarbones meet like a winged bird centred on a chest from which poke hard little teats. Ribs are slashes scored into her sides like gills. Between the portals of bent knees, the emerging child immediately establishes itself as the focus of the composition, the languid, doggy-paddling hands on either side of his head in complete contrast to the taut forms of the straining mother.

Sally stops in mid-sentence. 'What? Whose birth for God's sake?'

'The earth goddess Tlaz-ol-te-otl giving birth to the maize god.' I read the fine print on the reverse side. 'It's Aztec. Do you know it?' Sally is an artist. 'Remind me to show it to you next time you come over. There's something about it. It's – I don't know – kind of scary, kind of real. Elemental.'

The next time I see Sally is at her sister's house. Mina has just had her second child, a little girl, who is in her arms, plugged at her breast. Inevitably the conversation leads to the details of birth as experienced by the gaggle of women present. Home, hospital, doctor, midwife, Caesarean, birthing suite, drugs, enemas, episiotomies, candles, water baths, placenta stews, the usual. There is an undercurrent of one-upmanship about the degree of naturalness each mother has managed to achieve. I shrug off my loser position, having scored two emergency, highly medicalised Caesareans out of two births.

'My sons are no different from any other children for having used the trapdoor,' I assert. 'I watched this lady on the box having a baby in a rock pool in the manner of an ancient Polynesian or something – it's all the rage, capturing unusual births on video – and I kept thinking, that's all very well and good, except that out of camera range there's a good old Western doctor waiting to check on the mother and child. It's this selective plundering of cultures we deem more natural than our own that drives me wild . . .' This is a topic that once I start on I cannot stop. I jab my finger in the air. 'There is no such thing as "natural", according to anthropologists. All births are cultural, medical, technological. It's just different technologies, different cultures. We should either be Polynesians or not. I don't think we can take what we want from people with such impunity. I think it should be more difficult than that.'

The others know better than to engage me when I go off like this. Suddenly, pointedly, the baby needs attention. Babygros and organic baby soaps and potions and tying cocoons must be examined. To tell the truth, I'm just as sick and tired of my opinions. Like all strong views, they're defensive, catching me in a web of my own making. Why, only a few hours earlier that day I had again been thinking about that Aztec image on the postcard. Does the fact that I can respond to a statue from 1450 made by a remote and largely unfathomable society mean I should be willing to take on human sacrifice? What about the Polynesian-style rock pool birth? The baby had floated out from between the mother's legs, white, semi-liquid, like a poached egg. It had swum underwater for a number of long seconds, nudged unhurriedly by the attending father as if he was already showing off his son's swimming skills. Then into his arms he lifted the unperturbed baby still tethered to his mother by the cord, a chalaza snaking through the brine.

'It reminds me of this thing Sam would say when he was

little.' I'm in conversation with Sally again, over tea. 'Out of the blue he'd look up at us with that earnest look on his face and say, "I was born in the sea and my daddy saved me." A number of times Sam said that to us. Can you believe it! Weird, huh? We asked him "What? Where?" but he didn't have an answer. We never got to the bottom of it. I thought he was remembering something that had happened at the beach with Paul, but the temptation is there to think that he's remembering something about his birth. Except . . .'

Sally winces. 'It would have been fresh on his mind, being only – what?'

'I'm serious. Two and a half, three. Except, Paul wasn't there when he was born.'

Through the steam rising from our green tea, a picture wells up: Paul is avoiding me, looking at the monitor that is attached via a looping bundle of wires (a chalaza) through my body to the scalp of the stuck baby. Meconium in the water. Foetal distress. Emergency. Panic. No time or place for the father in the operating theatre. I fetch Linda's postcard to show Sally. We pore over Tlazolteotl.

'It's the squatting versus legs-in-the-stirrup, on-your-back-thing,' Sally says. 'This is the definitive position.'

'On your toes?'

'It's only a moment in time. As soon as the amazing maize god' – we guffaw – 'is out, she can flop back.'

In the narrative of a life, the birth of a child soon becomes subsumed by the streams and streams of moments thereafter. The endless number of repetitive tasks that follow, the long chains of nights and days lull one into forgetting, forgetting even the one event that started it all. But when the split second becomes forever, hardened in stone or caught by a camera – as Muybridge discovered of galloping horses, *Look, they float!* – the results are astonishing. I suddenly remember another incident when the boys were small. There are my two trapdoor boys, heads bent over, giggling, stabbing fingers into a hidden amusement, their voices weaving together into grunting snorts and explosive jingles. Intense curiosity disguised as a casual glance over their heads identifies the source of such furtive fun. It's a photograph in a book I had left around for them to find, believing it was good for them. What has them entranced is not the moony, glowing, colour images of the developing foetus in the womb (fish – fowl – baby), but a black-and-white snapshot of that moment when the mother is speared to the bed, flat on her back, Western style, and the baby's head is impossibly emerging from that strange place.

I dig up the book from inside a cardboard box in the garage. The binding is splitting and the book opens at the place of its own accord – perhaps the image has been revisited many times more than I know. The photograph that straddles the gutter is now in two separate pieces. In some way this adds to the feeling of mismatching fracture that the forms elicit.

The mother is a two-being, her body pulled apart in an ownership tussle. From her end, the baby's head is a surprising eruption from down below. The shock-white pallor of her exhausted face says, 'Who is this? Who am I?' Shift your head to the right and the baby is in ascendancy. His creased cry is as assertive as a cock's crow, the mother's splayed legs a set of powerful shoulders for him, her fine pubic hairs a decorative ruff on the V-neck of a now-it's-there, now-it's-not garment. The battle rages over the thickened torso. It see-saws between them on its belly button fulcrum. Blink once and the mother gains the upper hand, look again and the micro-headed baby is the victor.

It's Tlazolteotl giving birth to the maize god in a different context. The cultural frame is up to date, a softened, modified hospital birth with the father present, his arms encouragingly draped across his wife's shoulders as the head is delivered. He is radiant, beaming, as he watches his progeny emerge. At the foot of the bed the midwife, her elbow casually resting on the mother's thigh, waits to catch the baby. Tlazolteotl's lonely, elemental battle to deliver her son in stone is translated into flesh and caring. Art turned into life? Gods turned into people? In essence they are the same.

'It *is* highly amusing,' I say to Beryl, who has come to borrow a lawnmower and ends up staying for a chat while her teenage daughter hangs out with the boys in the band practice room. The book lies open near the postcard on the kitchen table.

'A push-me, pull-you toy, bloody funny. A rude picture, nothing glamorous. No soft focus, no baby advert here,' she says. 'Kids recognise that this is the bare truth and it's pretty weird. Also, I think they sense what no one will openly admit. A bit of the mother has to die so that this new person can live. I mean, you can't tell me that a new person is made out of all that healthy food you ingest when you're pregnant – liver and greens and stuff. It's the mother that is being gobbled up and transformed to make the baby. It's physics, isn't it?'

This is what I appreciate about Beryl. She says things that are *not nice*.

'I don't think kids have the capacity to sense that,' I counter. 'They're too egocentric to notice or to care.'

'Maybe, but every woman I know complains of it. Your hair falls out, your teeth rot. Your body is never the same. And as for the brain drain! Brain cells are actually lost when you're pregnant or around young children, no doubt about that. The only question is whether the damage is permanent,' she muses.

'Don't forget the lawnmower,' I remind her as she leaves with her daughter in belly-revealing tow. We laugh.

I think the earth goddess knows what Beryl has said to be true. She might be a major goddess in the Aztec hierarchy, but post-partum she senses a sea change. The balance of power is tipped. Without her maize offspring, her subjects are goners, this she acknowledges. Even if she does not fully comprehend it at the moment of his birth, submerged as she is in her own body, her own pain, she soon will. The expression on the maize god's face as he is born from her is that of a child who is being thwarted – denied a treat at the café sweet counter – or a man whose wife has served him a burnt meal. His gloomy, down-turned mouth speaks of sulks and tempers, a haughty manner with high expectations. He flaps his hands in the air. 'You really think this will do?' he says in sarcasm-loaded Aztec. I know once she is rocked back off her stony tiptoes, flopped down in exhaustion after the delivery, the earth goddess will soon harness what little strength she has left and do the things mothers and wives do: feed her baby, get up, soothe, make good.

'You came out looking like your father with a headache from doing the income tax return,' my mother has told me many times. 'Your head was as large as a football. I pushed and pushed and pushed but nothing doing. They yanked you out with forceps and when I saw your face it was all squashed.'

I'm lounging on Norma's sofa when I continue with this train of thought. 'I've been thinking of my traumatic birth. Do you remember in the sixties or seventies when primal screaming was all the rage? I had a friend, David Bernstein, who got himself all the way to Los Angeles to do the therapy with the founder . . . What was his name? Janosch? Something like that – it will come back to me in a second. Anyway, you spent days screaming, crying, clawing your way through your mother's birth canal so that you could be healed. It's laughable, yet . . .'

Norma is nodding her head vigorously. As an American she is all too eager to talk therapy.

'. . . yet it's got to be at the heart of things, the manner in which one is born. It sets the tone for life.'

This is all that it takes to get Norma going. She rattles on for a good hour about current available therapies that address the issue from different perspectives, as if she's quoting the latest consumer survey of home appliances. While she talks, I think of myself and my two boys and our struggles – could they be the result of three decidedly un-Polynesian birth experiences? – and these thoughts make me so uncomfortable I need to leave. My ears are ringing with Norma's grinding accent.

When I return home, Maureen is standing tiptoe on the stepladder, cleaning the windows.

'What was it like when you were in the hospital giving birth to Mawabo?' I ask her.

'I pushed Mawabo out and I burst!' she tells me, this mother, barely five feet, two inches, having, as she likes to put it, already signed for her height. 'The stitches, oh, the stitches. They sewed me up inside and outside for hours and hours. When it was time for me to go home, I could hardly walk.'

'How did you manage with the baby and all?' I asked.

'I was no longer a child. I was a mother now, taking the pain. I must live life as two now, not one.'

The two-being, being a parent, is a permanent condition. Birth is not, despite all the therapies around. Although it might be the seminal moment in each of our lives, I cannot take it that seriously and neither, I see, does my friend Linda in Amsterdam.

After a couple of weeks, I clean up the kitchen table, starting afresh as one does, time and time again. I shut the splitting book of photographs and stuff it back on top of the nearest shelf, pick up the debris that litters the tabletop, heap it to one side and sponge down the oilcloth. Before dropping Linda's postcard into a drawer along with a useful rubber band, a homeowner's supplement that includes an advert for a skylight I wish we could afford, an electricity account and the metal thingamajig that holds mosquito coils, I read the scrawled message on the reverse side once again. (How I love Linda's loopy, loony script!)

Dear you

I saw this at the newspaper stand on the corner and for some strange reason I thought of you, my friend. It's something I don't and won't know. It's not pretty but it's the way (more or less) you brought those two lads into the world so I think it's worth thinking about every now and then. But not too often. Look at the sky, look at flowers, look at your handsome boys when they are being good or not so good. Put a leg out in the sun for me. Amsterdam is cold.

Love, Linda

Between Life and Dust

Mark Patrick

A young woman rushes into the emergency room. There is terror in her eyes. In her arms she carries a baby girl, warm but barely breathing. 'My baby is dying,' she says, the terror in her voice too. She can't be more than twenty.

I am the paediatrician in this emergency room. I call my wife, Jean, also a paediatrician, who is down the passage in her consulting room. And the nurse. I need help. Quickly.

The child is blue and breathes weakly. My wife arrives and starts putting up a drip.

The baby's pulse is fading. I give oxygen. Her throat is blocked with blood-stained mucus from her lungs.

I call: 'Laryngoscope!'

The nurse cold-thuds it into my hand.

'Tube. Suction.'

More blood and mucus from her throat.

My wife gives me the tube, which I insert into the child's windpipe. She tries to cough, but can't.

I call: 'Ambubag!'

Jean attaches the oxygen bag to the tube. I squeeze the bag, trying to breathe oxygen into the child's very sick lungs. Blood gasps up the breathing tube.

Again I see the terror in the young mother's eyes. 'My baby's going to die,' she says.

I try harder, squeeze harder to get oxygen into her baby's lungs. There is a sudden loss of pressure in the oxygen bag.

Oh God, there is blood in my wife's face. I see the problem. There is a crack in the connector between the oxygen bag and the breathing tube. I call for another oxygen bag: 'Ambubag!' My voice breaks.

But it is too late.

I have sprayed the child's lung-blood, aerosolised, into Jean's face and eyes. When I look up, her tears are already washing it away.

When I look down, I see the child is dying despite our life-support efforts. I turn to the child's mother. 'I'm so sorry,' I say. 'It's time to say goodbye.' She looks away, her body racked by sobs. I feel her anguish.

It echoes my own, when our last two pregnancies miscarried. Jean is pregnant now, with a hoped-for daughter. We call her Rosemary.

Jean is at the basin. Washing, flushing her eyes with lukewarm water.

Before I hand the child's body, still warm, to her mother for their last goodbye, I do an examination, hoping not to find the signs that Jean and I know will be there. The baby is thin and her muscles are wasted. Her glands are enlarged, everywhere. Her liver is big and her spleen is big. All are signs of HIV infection.

Jean stops flushing her eyes. But they remain wet. For a long time.

Jean and our unborn child are now exposed, substantially and significantly, to the virus, which neither my president nor my employer, the minister of health, believes in.

Jean leaves. I am wrenched between the mother of my unborn child and another mother, mother of my dead patient. I ask vain-hopefully: 'Have you ever had an HIV test?'

'Yes. But I don't know the result.'

She agrees that I test her baby's blood, and I send it to the hospital laboratory marked 'URGENT'. Jean goes to Casualty to get her post-exposure anti-retroviral prophylaxis AZT and 3TC.

Now there is a triple risk. Jean can get HIV. Our unborn child can get HIV. And the effects of AZT and 3TC in pregnancy are unknown.

I cannot wait for the 'URGENT' test. With strangled hope and head in hand, I open my patient's folders. Four months ago, the dead child's mother came to my hospital for her antenatal check. Yes, she was tested for HIV. No, there is no record in the folders of the test result, nor of pre- or post-test HIV counselling. She went home.

Maybe it's negative, I tell myself, still clinging to vain hope.

I read on through the scanty, upside-down, shambled records. It doesn't take long.

One month later the mother came back and was admitted. She was bleeding and there were labour pains. She was only seven months pregnant. They tried to stop her bleeding and her contractions, but failed. She was transferred to a distant specialist hospital because of the pre-term labour, for her baby to be delivered early, by Caesarean section. They missed this opportunity to obtain her HIV test result, and to do HIV counselling. There is no further note in my patient's folders. Until today, when the baby died: 'Too sick to weigh, taken to ER.'

I phone the lab. I ask for the mother's result of four months ago. The telephone trembles in my hand.

'It's positive,' the technician says.

'And the baby's?' I ask. 'We sent it half an hour ago.' I know that it cannot be different, yet I hold on to the hope that it might be. I sprayed that blood into my wife's face.

'It's also positive.'

The mother does not know. Jean knows, without knowing, but like me she's hoping, even while swallowing her post-exposure anti-retrovirals.

Now what? Do I go to my wife or my patient? Who do I tell first? After all, the child's mother has been hoping too. Hoping but knowing, knowing but hoping, like the two paediatricians who'd been unable to save her baby's life.

It blurs. I go to Jean. I go to the bereft mother. I tell them both. The grieving woman knows.

I never see her again.

I drive home for lunch. On the radio it's *Midday Live*. The jaunty anchorman interviews the lawyer who advises our president on the non-existence of AIDS. I hear the lawyer saying that South African doctors are stupid. They have been hoodwinked by the pharmaceutical companies that manufacture AZT into thinking that there's such a thing as HIV killing people. No, he broadcasts, it's the AZT that kills. I stop my car and listen, slumped over the steering wheel. I cannot turn off the radio.

At home I go online. Searching with 'Ask Jeeves', I type *AZT 3TC first trimester*. I find a university site, where I can 'ask an expert'. I ask:

I am a paediatrician working in South Africa, the global centre of the pandemic. My wife is in the first trimester of our pregnancy. She has had HIV-infected blood splashed into her eyes, and is taking AZT and 3TC. What is the HIV infection risk to her and the foetus? What is the risk to the foetus of taking AZT and 3TC? Thank you.

I submit to cyberspace, and must wait.

I phone a colleague, an academic infectious diseases expert. The teratogenic effects of AZT and 3TC are unknown in early pregnancy. It would seem that the risk of damage to the unborn foetus is remote.

Jean phones her mother, who's also a doctor. She doesn't know.

Jean and I talk.

Tim, our first child, is healthy and strong. We have lost two pregnancies. AZT and 3TC reduce, but do not completely take away, the risk of HIV infection for Jean and our unborn child. AZT and 3TC may cause serious deformities as our foetus develops. But the risk is low.

We decide. We cannot take the risk. Jean and I are the only paediatricians serving a population of 1.2 million people. We are not strong enough to look after the desperately ill children entering our under-resourced health system and a seriously deformed child of our own. We decide to end Rosemary's short life.

Jean phones her doctor. Yes, we should do it. Yes, he'll do it. But not in the hospital where Tim was born, all bright colours, lights and smiling nurses. In the other one, where they do the terminations of pregnancy.

We drive for two hours to that place.

In the other hospital Jean, graduate-like, dons a grey gown. They take her, and Rosemary. I wait in the recovery room. It is dull, grey, cold. I remember what the Bible tells me, that I was born a sinner. I feel like a sinner now.

They wheel Jean back, no eye contact, no smile, no reassurance. The tears are still there, in her eyes and mine, the blood now between her legs. Rosemary is gone. We go. Furtively. Then to Granny's house. Granny is looking after Tim, too young to know that his sister is dead. Jean lies down. Granny comforts her. Tim is somewhere.

I stand alone next to the fridge. I see the crack where I tried to fix it once, instead depleting it of its coolant. And I buckle, before the white fridge door.

Not Yet a Mother

Tanya Wilson

This story is about a first birth, the only kind I know. Mostly it is a story about *not* knowing, and full of paradoxes, the first being that while birth is possibly the deepest and most powerful symbol in human existence, the actual experience of it could not be more devoid of symbolic thinking; it could not be more *concrete*. This has been particularly interesting – and at times alarming – for me, as thinking symbolically is a crucial component of psychoanalytic psychotherapy, a world that I had inhabited for some nine years before falling pregnant. In that world, birth represents, among other things, the union of mother and baby, but also the first rupture, the start of a lifelong journey in which we gradually separate into ourselves. In fact, on a symbolic level birth represents almost everything that psychoanalytic thinkers are interested in.

Yet for me, such symbolic thinking became harder as my pregnancy progressed. Previously, I would be quick to engage in the sleuth work of finding symbolic layers to people's stories, but I found that I became much more interested in facts and bodily realities for their own sakes. For example, I had been given a pre-birth gift of Margaret Wise Brown's famous children's book *Goodnight Moon*. This seemingly simple narrative, a variation on the universal maternal quest to settle a child to sleep, unfolds as a litany of saying goodnight to a range of objects in the child's surroundings. Gradually and peacefully, the bedroom darkens, the child falls asleep and the mother disappears from the bedside rocking chair. As clean and straightforward as its title suggests, this story perfectly satisfied my level of concreteness, although, as Joan Acocella points out in the *New Yorker* magazine, *Goodnight Moon* is ultimately a profound message from parent to child: *You don't want to go to sleep, I don't want to die, but we both have to.* But at the time I was not thinking like that any more, and together with my simplicity of mind came a corresponding cheerfulness, part of the deep sense of well-being that I was blessed with, particularly during the middle stage of pregnancy. I felt more content than I had ever known myself to feel. I was without anxiety or depression. I felt happy, but not excessively so. I felt *well*. It was not as if I did not get tired, but it was limited to physical tiredness, rather than the mixture of fatigue and existential conflict that I was more accustomed to. And it was a huge relief, as if I had been let off some indefinable hook.

An extraordinary feeling came over me at times: a mix of physical satisfaction and subtle emotion. It is a feeling that I have experienced on very rare occasions. I remembered having had it as a child, and was surprised by a childhood memory of having vaguely associated the words 'family feeling' with it. Physically, it is a state of deep contentedness; emotionally, it is a state of near-crying. It is something I had never spoken of, or named, or even consciously thought about. Yet its presence has persisted. Having the feeling again in relation to my unborn baby, I became aware that it must be associated with the intimate connectedness that human beings are capable of, the universality of human bonding.

Despite this effect of pregnancy, shadows of uncertainty and dread coexisted with my sense of well-being from the start. I had previously had what is known as an anembryonic pregnancy – a pregnancy with an embryonic sac, but no embryo; a miscarriage, but with no baby to mourn, only the fantasy to let go of. So, in addition to the expected nausea and exhaustion, the first few months aroused in me primitive images of loss and stagnation. This early stage also involved secrecy, as the prior experience had made me cautious about telling people that I was pregnant. A cherished secret is a magnet for private fantasies, and can be very effective at keeping reality at bay. As the second trimester approached, I became tense about the transition from my pregnancy being a private matter to it becoming public knowledge. I had worried about the absence of change; now I worried about the change itself. I was unspeakably anxious about telling my first client, but also nervous about telling others around me. Telling made it real, and its reality included an impending disruption to all my relationships at the time: husband, siblings, friends and, not least, clients. These worries resurfaced towards the end of my pregnancy. I remember thinking about the word 'impact' a lot. I thought of the sheer physical impact on me, and of the ripple effects that having a baby would produce within my professional and social world. And I thought about the fact that my impact on this baby would be greater than any I had made on anyone else, ever.

○

I did not know, when my waters broke around eight p.m. on the evening of 11 August 2005, that the birth of my first baby was to bring about a period of deep inner chaos: an unravelling – and gradual rethreading – of my very being. In fact, I was calm, and went to the bathroom to clean myself up before finding my husband to inform him – rather matter-of-factly, I think – of what had begun. My level-headedness continued while I talked to my midwife over the phone. After checking that I had had no contractions and that the water was not contaminated with meconium, she suggested that I try to get some sleep and that, if the labour did not progress, I should call her around seven the next morning. The underlying message was that I would be unlikely to go into full-blown labour that night.

I had told my midwife that there was no green meconium stain in the waters that broke, but as soon as I put down the phone I was gripped by doubt about this. Having flushed most of the fluid down the toilet, I became obsessed with checking my water-stained underwear over the course of the next hour, and each time it appeared to get greener and greener. At the same time I seemed unable to see colour, as though my brain had seized in that area of discrimination, and I could not trust my own eyes. I knew that meconium in the water was a danger sign, and already I was consumed by maternal concerns that I might misread clues essential to my baby's well-being.

Paralysed by my sudden incompetence, and feeling like a paper boat setting out on an unknown ocean, I did what I was told and went to bed. Of course it was impossible to sleep, and after futile attempts to read, I simply lay with my eyes open. The angles of our attic bedroom remained fixed and shadowed above me, and I listened to the sea moving slowly below. In the grey light the night sheds on our bedroom, with my husband fast asleep beside me, something began to happen. What I remember is a low-grade period pain, not enough to warrant getting out of bed. Some time later I was hit by waves of diarrhoea: each time there was a spasm I had to run to the toilet. I obeyed these physical urges several times, and wondered stupidly whether this was actually a gastric bug, a twenty-four-hour virus that was going to complicate the birth process. I was unconvinced that labour had really begun, and if it had, I was sure that the diarrhoea had nothing to do with it. My inability to see the obvious is laughable now, but I have subsequently discovered that I am not the only woman who has been so unsure of her own labour.

Is it powerful denial or is it in the nature of new experience that it is utterly different from the descriptions one has heard or read about? Something certainly happens when we are faced with an unfamiliar reality that clouds our capacity to place it. In retrospect I see these gaps in my own perceptions as evidence of the first strip being torn from the self that I knew. It was the first clue that the language of meaning I had built to understand my self and the world was profoundly lacking. I thought I knew something about birth and motherhood. I was aware that there were things I did not know, but I assumed that they would be things that would *add* to my knowledge in an interesting but ordered and manageable way, rather than in the manner of a bomb exploding.

In the past, women frequently died in childbirth, and I doubt that our evolutionary response has caught up with today's decreasing mortality statistics. Inside the heightening chaos of labour, I was caught between anxieties stemming from my sense of the danger of childbirth and the notion that one should summon medical professionals only when one is quite far into labour, so as not to waste their time. This apprehension was all the more loaded in the middle of the night, when things are never what they seem. Some time into the waves of abdominal spasms, I stopped returning to bed and started pacing the house. My husband, sensing my agitation, woke up and came down to be with me. I ended up spending much of this period of time in my unborn baby's room. This was totally unplanned, but the room was closest to the toilet and had a spare bed, where I made desperate but unsuccessful attempts to lie down and rest. There was also a carpet on which I could kneel on all fours, the most comfortable position for the contractions.

My husband's presence was essential – I would have been very frightened without it – but at the same time peripheral to the overwhelming reality of the contractions. By now I realised that they *were* contractions, probably because I no longer had to run to the toilet every time one came. But timing them was another matter. I couldn't decide at what point one started, or when it ended. On the one hand, they seemed to be there all the time; on the other, they did not seem to last long enough to warrant phoning the midwife. At two in the morning, prompted by seeing some blood in the toilet bowl, I finally pressed the numbers to wake her. As if to confirm that I was being feeble, my contractions abated while I talked to her, and I was hopelessly inadequate in describing them. But despite this, she surprised me by suggesting that we meet at the hospital. In previous discussions she had said that she would first come to our home. In fact, I had thought she might encourage a home birth. When she told me to meet her at the hospital, I felt two things simultaneously: pride that I had not phoned her too early, and fear that perhaps we were in an emergency.

We live on a mountainside above the coast. There are eighty-seven steep steps from the house down to where we park our car, and that does not include several landings (also at a gradient) between the steps. As I began the descent, I was deeply grateful that it was such an ungodly hour, for it meant that I would not be likely to meet any upbeat neighbours making their way up or down the stairs as I clutched the railing every few steps. It seemed to take hours to get down, and I longed to be in the car, rushing towards the hospital. But once in the car, constricted by the shape of the seat and strapped in by a seat belt, I was desperate to get out again. The only way to tolerate the horror that gripped my abdomen and lower back was to move, or to be on all fours, holding on to something solid and still. Sitting upright became the most ludicrous position, and I writhed around in my straitjacket, moaning and grasping whatever I could. There was one moment on the drive to the hospital that broke through the torture, a comic scene when, on the empty highway, we hurtled towards a solitary car and saw that it was my midwife, driving with perfect composure. Aware of the ridiculous picture we made, we sped past her, giving in to the illogical urgency of getting there first.

My husband dropped me at the hospital entrance, and once he had left to park the car, I gave in to a contraction. I have a vivid memory of the next few minutes of being alone, walking into the quietness of the hospital as though I were a visitor, my ordinary self restored, speaking calmly to the man at reception and then getting into the lift to go up to the maternity ward. As it happened, my midwife had already phoned the hospital, and the nurse on duty had been instructed to check on my baby's heart rate. Once again I had to be strapped in, this time lying on an adjustable bed that immediately felt like a dentist's chair, with a contraption over my abdomen to monitor the baby's heartbeat. As the contractions returned, I wanted to tear the monitor off and plead maltreatment. But I had been through this procedure before, just before my due date, to ensure that all was well with my baby's heart rate. I knew what it was for and how important it was. I also knew that it took longer than I would have liked.

My husband and midwife arrived together, reconfigured behind the scenes into a new team. Until the heart rate was established, everyone was tense. I watched their faces. On hearing that the heartbeat was normal, I relaxed a little. But my midwife had something else to check that would inform her of what kind of job lay ahead for her: the condition of my cervix, and how dilated I was. 'The moment of truth', she called it. And I understand why. Now I know how varied the birth process can be, that people can labour for more than twenty-four hours and not dilate beyond a few centimetres. Her examination would give some indication of not only what I was in for, but also what *she* was in for. I assumed at that point that I was still in for a long haul, that the level of pain would increase dramatically and that I would become more and more exhausted from it. My midwife started her examination. I watched her face like a baby watching its mother. There was that composure again, that deliberation, the hint of someone making sure of something; then a smile and some words. I don't remember them all, but I remember the phrase 'dream cervix' and a pleased 'six centimetres dilated'. I felt triumphant.

I did not notice at the time, but the so-called natural birth room looked like something in a Holiday Inn – plain and comfortable but devoid of taste: a king-size bed with no frills, a chair, perhaps some other furniture. Most significant was a huge bath on one side of the room. My midwife filled it for me and began putting sheets of manila paper, the kind I remember drawing on in pre-school, all over the floor. I climbed into the bath and was overwhelmed by relief as I lowered myself into the hot water. It was like sinking into myself. I was in safe hands. Someone who *knew* was going to stay with me until this was over. I could abandon the hyper-vigilance, the searching of faces. I was here: completely present in my body.

What followed was perhaps the wildest part of the birth for me. It was far from the image, commonly used in the media, of a woman pushing with every shred of her being to get her baby out. I was lying in the bath in a trance-like state. My contractions were frequent and crippling. But it is not the agony that I remember. I remember feeling hot and heavy and limp, like a large, wounded beast. I remember not being able to keep my eyes open. And in those moments between contractions, as I sank into myself, with a vague awareness of the two people tending me, as though they were a different species altogether, all human thought within me came to a stop.

In her calm and deeply containing way, my midwife knew before I did that I was getting ready to push, and that it would be easier to push if I was out of the bath. She got me to squat on the sea of paper on the floor, my back against the bed, with my husband sitting on the bed behind me, holding me under my arms. As the contractions came she told me to push. For once in this process, I really knew what to do; every fibre in me was poised for this. And so I pushed. Again. Again. Again. Again. On it went. On and on. My thighs began to burn, then to tremble and finally to shake uncontrollably. My midwife got me on to the bed and called the hospital midwife on duty. Again my husband held me from behind, while each of my feet was raised against the upper arms of the two midwives. They pushed against me; I pushed against them. My baby's head began to emerge between my thighs but I could not push it through. For what seemed like hours the head felt stuck there. I had somehow expected that it would retreat into the birth canal again while I mustered up the effort to push some more. But it did not; it stayed where it was. It was intolerable. It was one thing to push with my pelvis intact, but pushing while I was already split open felt impossible. I lost track of the contractions and could not tell when they were coming, or when to push. I swore. I bit my husband. I said, 'I can't do this,' over and over. Everyone disagreed. On it went. At this point my midwife was testing the baby's heartbeat after every push. I could hear her and the other midwife conferring. They were getting more agitated. The heart rate was dropping. I was losing my strength. I remember my midwife saying to me that if she made the tiniest cut, the head would slip out. Part of me wanted her to, so I didn't have to keep going myself. But on I went and, finally, the baby slid free. Out it came, slippery as a fish, caught by both myself and the midwife. I lifted it up to discover a girl. Oh, my baby.

Hannah. Here you are. You have come. We are cutting your cord. You are crying, but my first thought is that you do not seem overwhelmed. Let me hold you. That's it. The placenta that has sustained you these nine months is slipping out, as you just did.

You have already shown the way. Let us go to the bath. You can lie on me, and your father can cover you with a towel and pour warm water from the bath over it to keep you weighted and warm. Your body is complete. You have your arms and legs; your fingers and toes are curling. And your mouth, like a tiny sea anemone, is already suctioning, planting miniature kisses on my chest, searching, searching . . .

I felt an overwhelming sense of joy as I lay in the bath with Hannah on my chest, and a profound delight in my new knowledge of what it was to give birth. Part of the relief when it was over was the sense that I had an account, a progression, a story that I could tell. Of course, I had no idea that the story was not over, far from it. It was Hannah's birth that was over; my own birth, my psychological birth as a mother, had not yet begun.

ℂ

I did not know just how much I would falter, post-birth, without the symbolic space that I had become accustomed to as a psychotherapist. As much as my departure from symbolic thinking felt like a reprieve when I was pregnant, so it became more frightening after Hannah's birth. During her birth, I was given a hint of what it is like to be in a place in which one has no sense of direction, no road signs and, most frightening, no way even of marshalling one's own thoughts. Some two months afterwards, this experience of deep inner chaos began to dominate. I could not sleep; I was anxious and forgetful; I was unable to name or place things; I could only grasp at memories of myself, like puddles of oil on water. Far from feeling let off the hook, as I had done during pregnancy, I became acutely aware that in fact now I *was* the hook. I was the hook that Hannah would attach to most powerfully. I was the mother, that most written-about figure in psychoanalysis, perhaps anywhere. The change was so enormous I simply could not *think* about it. Its impact was visceral. It would be some time before I realised that this sojourn outside symbolic space was a necessary part of the profound internal restructuring that would allow me to make something of my own out of what it is to become a mother.

○

Next to death, birth is the ultimate transition. How each of us responds to and deals with change is as unique as our fingerprints. I am struck by the fact that my first spontaneous thought about Hannah was precisely about her maiden transition, and about how easily she accepted it, although I do not assume that this is how change will always be for her. Only she can tell her story, in time. The story I can tell is something about my own transformation. For me Hannah's birth stays poised in the midst of it, in a place I can never return to, for I was not yet a mother at the time. Those eight hours, painful and chaotic as they were, remain indescribably gratifying in my memory. They were hours in which – safely held by those around me – I left the world of human symbols, the realm of existence as I knew it, and entered the realm of existence as it is. And, without thinking, I gave birth to my daughter – she who would sustain me on my re-entry, and in all the years ahead.

Doing It by the Book

Joanne Hichens

It's a Friday evening: 17 July 1993. I'm glued to *The Bold and the Beautiful*. My waters don't break, but I know this is it. I suffer the first twinges and shooting pains in my groin, then the hard knock of a knee or an elbow at my pelvis, a sharp jabbing at my gut. Jessica is flexing her muscles, letting me know she wants out. I've been told it's a girl. At one of my later scans, when she was dancing about in there, under my skin, the doctor got a clear view of what was between her legs, and it was no penis.

Brooke Forrester and I will be having our babies together, though Brooke's kid is likely to be three years old by the time I leave the hospital with my newborn.

I time six-minute intervals between contractions. 'We have to go, *now now now!*' I shriek at Robert, who is hiding out in some corner of our Mowbray semi, as I haul myself up the stairs to the bedroom and start cramming stuff into a suitcase. And so, too, starts the second-guessing, the rehashing. Am I ready for this? Is there last-minute studying I need to do? Do I need to brush up on birthing facts? Should I cross my legs and hold on a few more days so that I can practise my breathing and nappy-changing technique? Memorise top tips for breastfeeding? Do I have lanolin to protect nipples and lips and baby's bum? I cross-check against my list, several pages long, for wipes, nappies, suits and booties for the baby. Also, *not* to be forgotten, the cap knitted by Grandmother, with the pink pompom on top. Make-up, hairbrush, chocolates and magazines, eight pairs of big beige panties and plenty of super-absorbent stick-on sanitary towels.

Robert, hovering in the doorway, looks at me in much the same bemused way I'd been watching my soap, as if *I* am a soapie star, coming loose at the seams. 'Robert,' I say, in a last-minute panic, pulling from my suitcase a cotton dressing-gown the same dark pink of the areolas and vaginas and newborns illustrated in *the book*, 'I will not be seen in the passages of the hospital in this tatty old thing!'

Robert sighs, knowing better than to argue. He sits on the packed suitcase. I clamp it shut. He chauffeurs me to the mall where, between contractions, I try on the various styles of gown he brings me. 'I don't want beige or pink,' I say. 'Nothing fleshy.' Finally, I buy something blue and big as the ocean, from the Woolworths men's department. I choose a pair of fluffy slippers, too. Robert pays. He makes no comment. I am the one with the Bump. And after all, I have read *the book*. He has not.

The book says, *Only 5 per cent of babies arrive on their due date.* I know that's today, and so does Jessica.

Now we are ready.

○

I'm one of those perfectionists who do things 'right' in their head. In my head everything is planned to the last detail. But I find life, with all the choices it offers, so overwhelming that when it comes down to implementing my plans, I leave most things till the last minute. That way, I'm not responsible for imperfection. I'm off the hook! For instance, I've collected piles of photographs of my children, but I've never found the 'right' albums to stick them in, so they lie about gathering dust and fading in the sun. I organised my wedding, but fell short of getting the dress until the day before. In wedding photos I look as if a skyful of cumulus clouds has settled on my sleeves: of course, the 'perfect' dress at Meyers – stylish, elegant, off-the-shoulder – got sold to a more organised bride while I was trying to find the *most* perfect dress.

Birth, though, I swore I would be prepared for. And I was. I had read *the book*, several times over in fact. I'd referenced it the way fundamentalist Christians turn the pages of the Bible for guidance. I was relying on it to get me and Jessica through to the other side of birth. Of course, I skipped the parts that had to do with *home confinement, water birth, midwifery*. No alternative stuff for me. The baby would be delivered in the hospital, no question. I wanted to hear a healthy cry as the experienced and well-respected obstetrician/gynaecologist smacked Jessica on the bum and handed her over to the paediatrician to check from top to toe.

But my suitcase wasn't packed. I should have known then that I was about to do this birth the way I do most things. Imperfectly.

My mother still tells me stories about her miscarriage, blamed on an incompetent cervix. When she was pregnant with me, her doctor sewed in a Shirodkar stitch and pulled her uterus closed like a draw-string purse to keep me from falling into her vagina. The stitches became embedded in her flesh and couldn't be released, so, when I decided to make my way out, I couldn't move. It didn't help having the umbilical cord around my neck. At the last minute the beginner doctor was sacked and a specialist was called in to perform an emergency Caesarean section and release me from the stranglehold of death. 'You nearly killed me!' is my mother's punch-line, as she tells the story of the novice doctor who couldn't cope.

I wasn't taking any chances. I had found myself a doctor who came highly recommended, along with an anaesthetist and paediatrician who between them had qualifications from prestigious universities and years of baby-catching practice.

On my first visit to Dr R., once the pleasantries were done – the handshaking, the weighing, the chit-chat, the peeing in the pot – I lay with my legs spread while her gloved fingers felt for the signs and duration of pregnancy. I checked out her framed-in-gold degrees on the walls of her examining room, her scanning machine, her tissues and spatulas and probes. (How thoughtful she was to have pink and purple gowns in different sizes hanging from the back of the door.) I smiled as she palpated my abdomen, *detecting the general softening of the genital organs and the increase in the size of the uterus,* just as *the book* explained she would. I had got this right. I had chosen the perfect doctor.

Parentcraft classes should begin at this stage, said *the book,* so at six months I pulled Robert along to our evening sessions, where I diligently took notes and memorised facts as if birth was an exam I'd score an A+ for. This time, I would not stuff up. I would not leave studying till the last minute.

At parent classes we played with dolls. We practised folding cloth nappies and securing them with safety pins, even though I'd accumulated a stack of disposables in the cupboard at home. (I did not own up to this.) We bathed the dolls, we held them, we played mommy and daddy. I sneaked peeks at nervous moms-to-be, chewing their lips, biting their nails, and I patted myself on the back. No way could they have read as many books as I had: books on babies in the womb, antenatal care, post-natal care, child care, creative parenting. In between watching TV soaps and reading thrillers, I was studying child psychology and getting distinctions! I had gleaned tips on how to select a safe baby car seat, how to deal with swallowed objects and near-drowning. I knew how to travel long distances with children, and how to cope with divorce. Not only did I know about pregnancy and birth, but I knew which week to expect baby's first smile, her first incisors, her first word – 'Mama', no doubt.

At home, I sat cross-legged on a mat and worked on my Lamaze breathing patterns – *training my mind to respond to different types of contractions* – while I watched documentaries to come to terms with the reality of the baby's head crowning. I was both fascinated and repulsed by the bulging of the anus and the perineum as the uterine muscles pushed the baby out, the head showing through the slit of the stretching vagina, then slipping back. As if that particular baby had a sense of the state of the world and retreated into the womb, digging in its heels.

I remember, as a child, asking my mother, 'How does a baby get in there? Does it hurt when it comes out?' Later, in my teens, the only book that fascinated me as much as the illustrated guide to pregnancy and childbirth my mother gave me to study was a book my brother was given, on shark attacks. The middle section had gory full-colour pics of the chomped and bloodied thighs and calves of young men who'd undergone a different sort of life-changing experience.

172

I will not be squeamish, I told myself. This is the natural order of things. My vagina, too, will stretch to reveal a big-eyed clone. I will not, however, eat the placenta, though I had read that it could be *sautéed with onions to make a rather tasty dish, rich in iron.*

Now, on the highway, I frantically turn the pages of *the book*, checking on last-minute details, making sure I'm ready for the test. I'm on the verge of tears as I acknowledge somewhere within me the fragile line between the perfect birth and some of the scarier possibilities. Headings like *Emergency Caesar, Post-partum haemorrhage* and *Stillbirth* catch my eye.

I read aloud: '*The prepared husband should offer bananas, fruit juice and honey to his wife during labour. Offer small nibbles and sips, keep her hydrated and keep her energy levels up.*'

'Don't worry, I know my stuff,' Robert says, pulling in sharply at Waglay's Café, nearly denting the car as he bounces off the kerb.

'Jesus, Robert, calm down!'

'We have to hurry. No time to waste. We have to get to Vincent Pallotti in good time. One last stop, OK? For extra provisions. Just in case.' He squeezes my hand and says, '*If she swears and bites, don't take it personally!*'

'So, you've dipped into *the book* after all?' I squeeze his hand back, feeling more confident than ever, and grateful that my spouse has gone as far as reading the birth manual. He'd sympathised as I'd suffered bleeding gums, constipation, cramps and cravings. He'd suffered *The Bold, Days, All My Children.* I'd ordered him around for months, just as Brooke had ordered Ridge to do her every bidding. And Robert had complied. He had gone meekly to the Seven Eleven minutes before closing time to buy Cote d'Or Bouchées and soda water. (Thank God I never wanted to eat coal.)

Once, I spread myself on a chaise longue in our tiny garden, soaking up some winter sun and snapping my fingers, just as Brooke Forrester might have done, for Robert to bring me a cooldrink. Then I read that *sun will aggravate any pigmentation caused by the increased production of MSH (melonacyte stimulating hormone).* To avoid a rash of freckles, I went back to watching soaps in a darkened room.

As Robert puts a load of chips, Cokes, Liqui-Fruits and chocolate bars on the counter, the café owner asks, 'Are you going camping?'

'We're going to have our baby!' Robert beams. I turn to show off my bump, specially adorned for this auspicious event in an acrylic-mix twinset with faux pearl buttons.

'So this is your first, eh?' the café owner smiles.

'We want to be prepared for a long night,' Robert says.

The café owner nods and says, 'Mmm . . .', as if he knows something we don't.

'What did he mean by "Are we having our first?"?' I say, back in the car, a slight paranoia setting in that perhaps I don't know as much as I think I do.

'We know our stuff. Don't worry,' says Robert, patting my shoulder, the closest he can get to me physically these days.

I snap the medical-aid card between my fingers. I sit a little straighter. Back in control. Breathing deeply. Focusing on the kaleidoscope of colour behind closed lids. Then opening my eyes and blinking rapidly with the pain of another contraction. I'm impatient to get it all done with. Pop the kid. Pay the bill. This birth thing will be a breeze. I place *the book* on my knees and press my palms on the covers. This well-worn manual, with its dog-eared corners and stains of spinach and melted cheese on the pages I'd pored over during meals, is closed. I've done my homework. I've done all I can. It's too late now to do a thing more.

☉

Paperwork signed and clip-boarded, we are admitted to our room in the labour ward. Robert goes straight to work.

Bring a touch of home to the labour ward.

He unrolls a small carpet, soft under bare feet, and plugs in our lamp with its pale blue shade and a low-wattage bulb for gentle lighting. He sets up an aromatherapy lamp, lit from the inside by candles, and the soothing fragrance of lavender oil fills the room. I insist on wearing my own clothes to start with, and change into a flared tracksuit top.

'Robert, cover those items over there,' I command. He throws a sheet over an array of tools laid out on a trolley: vacuum machines, tubes and timers, round-tipped scissors and pointy ones, and scalpels.

That's better, the green sheet less ominous than the glint of light on steel. And Dr R. will not need any of that metal for this birth. I will not be opened like a tin can to have my baby scooped out. I am going to push, after all, like any normal woman. I will squat and walk and breathe and push, just as *the book* has described I should, and the baby will drop neatly into the world.

Robert rigs up our portable TV and plugs in M-Net.

'What's on tonight? Have you checked the TV guide?'

'Just rubbish for now.' So we play Scrabble between contractions and shallow breathing. I nibble on energy foods, joking around to see which birth words we can lay out – *natural, joyful, supermom* – while avoiding words like *forceps, pethidine, episiotomy, faeces*. We play until one particularly strong contraction sends the board flying. (We never found every piece, and so to this day we are limited to spelling words that exclude the letter *q*.)

Robert grips my hand at the height of another intense contraction. I puke up morsels of banana and honey. So much for those snacks intended to keep up my energy.

'I need a bath,' I announce. I need to clean up, to regain my composure. So I languish, whining and half delirious, till the bathwater turns lukewarm and globs of blood float and spiral under the surface. Some other poor sod bangs on the door demanding her turn, and reluctantly I get out. My top now replaced with standard-issue hospital gear, I waddle down the passage with the stays of the garment untied, not caring who gawps at my bare buttocks swaying about as I moan my way back to the labour ward.

'Turn off the TV!' I shriek as I haul myself back into bed.

'Is this movie any good, Robert?' Dr R. says, as John Wayne gallops across the screen, guns blazing.

'You're supposed to be helping me, not watching some crappy Western!' I shout. 'My back is killing me! When will this baby come? Ooergh!' I sound like a truck with brakes on, screeching down a sixty-degree hill.

'You have the pain threshold of a man,' Robert says.

'What happened to *never criticise, use positive phrases if you can*, Robert?'

'Can you keep it down a little?' he says. 'You know three centimetres isn't classified as real labour, right? That's what *the book* says.'

'Robert,' I reply, seething, 'one more word and I'm gonna take those braai tongs from under that green sheet over there and rip your goddamned tongue from your throat! And will someone turn on the lights in here? Stuff the soft lighting! Someone, anyone, look up my vagina, for god's sake, and ask this baby when she's coming out! Tell her to come! Now!'

Robert takes a call on the payphone outside the labour ward. 'It's your mother,' he tells me. 'She says she can hear you shrieking up there in Pretoria!'

The lavender in the incense burner clogs my sinuses. The TV is still on, the crack of Colt .45 gunfire and my screams competing for Robert's attention. If I wasn't strapped down with the electronic foetal monitoring system, I'd take every prop and toss it through the plate-glass observation window. 'Give me the epidural! Now!' I yell.

There is no way Dr R. dare refuse, though the nurses tell me I've progressed nicely, to at least four centimetres dilated. *As the baby's head is delivered, it will feel like toothpaste being squeezed from a tube*. But who knows how long it will take to reach that magic measurement of ten centimetres when the baby will glide out?

'It may take three hours, it may take six,' Dr R. tries to explain. As I beg for relief, the nurses nervously approach to check the graphs.

'This cannot be childbirth! This is torture! And what happened to wiping my face, massaging my back, holding my hands, eh?' I ask Robert, his jaws working mechanically through packet after packet of chips.

At last, I sit on the edge of the bed, my heaving belly in front of me. I spew bile into a kidney-shaped silver dish as the spinal drip sinks in and, almost immediately, hallelujah, I can breathe again. And I don't feel a thing. I lie down, my legs bent and apart. I keep my eyes on the ceiling, wishing there was a Brueghel print up there, as at the dentist, so I can stare at sheep or milkmaids while the business happens down below. Meanwhile, Robert's eyes are nearly popping from his head as he watches the soapie unfolding right before him. He soon heads off to a safe distance and continues to munch on the supplies.

I don't know how many hours later it is that I reach the final moments of labour. There is no way I can push. My legs are numb. *But who cares?* The nurse whips the sheet off the collection of instruments that remind me of the scrambled utensils in my kitchen drawer. Dr R. can extract the baby with whatever she wants to, as long as I don't feel a thing.

At last Dr R. hands me Jessica, her eyes blinking through vernix, a small brush of bruising on the sides of her head where the forceps were clamped on her skull to yank her out. I love my daughter at first sight. But I am able to admire her small, creased face for only a second or two before a nurse whips her away and I lie, spent, to eject the placenta. Then, cleaned up and sewn up, I am wheeled away from the torture chamber to my room, where I sleep a good number of hours till another nurse brings her back to me.

○

I was a guest in hospital for three days, alternately suffering exhaustion, love, irritability, hospital meat as tasty as cardboard, and sloppy jelly and custard. Nurses with no permission pinched my nipples to squeeze out colostrum and so tempt my daughter to latch on. For three days I smelled like a poorhouse as I cooked cabbage on my engorged, hotplate breasts. I pulled out limp leaf after leaf from my double-D-cup beige nursing bra, which matched the very large beige panties accommodating those giant pads. In the first few photos of me and Jessica, somewhere in that pile at home, I look exhausted, with strands of sweaty hair plastered across my forehead.

On my hospital TV, Brooke languished in bed in her silk shorty pyjamas, her sleek hair brushed into a ponytail. She was bright-eyed with make-up *au naturel*, looking as though she was about to hop out of bed and head for her aerobics class. A couple of episodes later, while I rubbed cream into my sore, cracked nipples, I watched Brooke drop off her kid at kindergarten. The child had skipped the terrible twos. She'd had no tantrums. She had a mouthful of pearly whites and a Spanish nanny trailing after her, while Mommy fooled around and most likely got herself pregnant again, with her – now ex-husband's – father or brother or cousin.

Thank God for ice packs and salt baths to soothe the vagina. Within a few days, my wounds were on the mend and I was limping about, getting back to normal (if there is such a thing as 'normal' after having children).

As I packed to leave the hospital, I discovered a Shoprite plastic bag under my bed. 'That's your placenta to take home,' the nurse said. She suggested I feed my garden with it, but the closest I come to gardening is buying a bunch of roses from Woolworths, so I politely declined. I opted to take home only my suitcase and my baby, Jessica: this perfect child, our daughter, snug in her baby seat, her crowning glory the cap with the pink pompom.

Though I'm no longer hooked on *The Bold*, I know that Brooke Forrester is now a grandmother several times over, maybe even a great-grandmother, even though she still looks twenty-nine. Me, I have to go every six weeks to get my grey roots dyed. We've had two more children – Louise and Alister – and Robert has had a vasectomy. I don't know why, but I still have *the book* on my shelf.

Everything by Heart

Colleen Higgs

I was so much older than most first-time mothers-to-be. I wandered into bookshops and paged through countless books about babies, feeling like an impostor. The world of motherhood felt like a foreign country; I didn't belong to it, nor it to me. I was hoping for a story to guide me into this hinterland, to teach me its customs and folkways. Little did I know that I would have to learn everything by heart.

I gave scant attention to information in the pregnancy guides about possible complications in pregnancy, such as pre-eclampsia, out of a vague superstition that my full attention would only tempt fate. Pre-eclampsia is a potentially life-threatening condition for mother and child, which usually strikes late in pregnancy. Older mothers, especially those having their first baby, are more likely to develop it. Little is known about its causes or about possible preventive measures, partly because the window for studying it is very small, but the best treatment is to deliver the baby.

At twenty-nine weeks I thought I was having a stroke. I felt unbearably hot and nauseous, and the pain was excruciating – for some reason especially intense under my right rib. It was difficult to breathe, my skin felt too tight, I felt I might implode. All were symptoms of pre-eclampsia.

I realised in retrospect that there had been signs in my pregnancy that something was not right. I'd been ill and tired throughout the twenty-nine weeks, and had none of the positive symptoms described in the books. I'd had several serious migraines, the pain so severe it would make me vomit. All of these episodes were either on Sundays or public holidays, which meant house calls by the doctor and paying extra for the blissful relief of the three-in-one injection cocktail – Voltaren, tranquilliser and anti-nausea medication – that would ease the intense, prolonged pain and vomiting and finally bring sleep.

I was admitted to hospital on a Monday, and told by my gynaecologist/obstetrician, Dr J., that she would try to keep my baby girl inside me for as long as possible. I wore a belt across my chest to monitor her heartbeat. She seemed to be doing OK. After the third pre-eclampsia episode, Dr J. decided to do an emergency Caesar on the Thursday – 30 May 2002 – which would make my baby eleven weeks early. When I first realised that she was going to be premature, that I was unable to incubate her inside my body where she belonged, I cried with guilt and sadness, feeling that I had let her down.

At the delivery, André, my husband, was at my head with the anaesthetist, while the lower half of my body was hidden behind a curtain. Being very tall, André could see over the screen and witnessed the entire procedure, from Dr J. cutting me open to the extraordinary moment when she pulled the tiny, bloody creature out. She looked nothing like the pictures of newborn babies in the books. She was tiny, almost fleshless, like a newly hatched bird that belonged firmly in its nest. She seemed old and wise, unearthly. My entire being flooded with tenderness as I held and kissed her for a few seconds before she was taken away from me. André followed her and the paediatrician out of the room to the neonatal intensive care unit (NICU). I saw her again only hours later, in the early evening. We named her Kate.

It's easy enough now to give a factual account of what I experienced in hospital, but it's not so easy to write about the inside of the experience, even less so to convey anything of what it might have been like for Kate. She underwent numerous blood tests in the form of pinpricks to her heels; she received several doses of antibiotics, iron drops to ward off anaemia, caffeine drops to make her heart beat faster, and oxygen too, although she didn't ever have to be on a ventilator. She had jaundice and spent three days and nights under UV lights in the first week of her life. She was given Surfactin to strengthen her lungs. She weighed only 1080 grams when she was born and then her weight dropped down to under a kilogram for a week or two.

The first day or so of Kate's life I felt sore from the Caesar, and my neck was painfully stiff from leaning over the incubator, and from the tension of the whole experience. My breasts were enormous and tender, and the only relief I got was from expressing my milk, which was pale brown when it first came in. At once it was sent off to the lab to be tested in case there was something wrong with it. I was ashamed as I waited for the results, unsure of myself, of my milk, of my role. When the lab determined that it was fit for Kate's consumption, I was relieved, filled with joy. I had dreaded the worst. She was initially given one ml at a time from a tiny syringe that was suspended cleverly above her with an elastic band and led into a tube down her nose straight into her stomach. I became adept at filling the syringe, at feeding my baby.

In the first ten days or so she lay in plain sight in an elevated open incubator against the back wall of the NICU. She was kept warm by the heated incubator and covered with a miniature space blanket when she wasn't being held. She was naked except for a tiny nappy and a great number of tubes and monitors attached to her body. She seldom cried, but when she did it was a peculiar sheep-like bleat.

One morning, while sitting in the plastic chair next to the incubator holding her next to my skin, I looked down at her and noticed that she had turned very white, almost blue. She was cold, too. Time stopped for me. The paediatrician was called and she was given a life-saving blood transfusion. I can't remember what it felt like to be in the moment of that ordeal. I have forgotten how hard it was. At the time, I coped by taking everything one day at a time, one hour at a time. I didn't plan or think ahead about next week or next month, or the end of my maternity leave.

While in the NICU, I watched other mothers who skilfully changed nappies and used special cotton buds and lotions and wipes. I hadn't bought anything for my baby, not wanting to tempt fate. While we were in hospital, André did the first baby shopping: prem nappies and Kate's first toy, a small, soft, purple Eeyore. I was shell-shocked, unprepared. It was enough witnessing her incubation from the outside. With the help of nurses, the paediatrician and other mothers, but mostly just by watching her closely, I began to figure out what she needed minute by minute. And what I was able to do.

Kate's birth brought an overflow of gifts: babygros, vests – even an embroidered one – hats, blankets, hand-knitted jerseys, booties, dungarees, miniature sheepskin slippers, a plastic bath chair, a pram, a cot and a house full of flowers.

I remember sitting in the NICU next to the incubator drinking tea about a week after Kate was born when the convener of the antenatal classes phoned to tell me that the date of the first meeting was postponed. At first I didn't know what she was talking about, then I started to cry. 'My baby has been born already,' I told her. She was sympathetic, which made me cry even more.

The first night I had to leave Kate in the hospital and go home was particularly bleak, the world wet and cold, the drive up Hospital Bend to Woodstock too far. My whole being resisted leaving, my arms felt empty, too light. For two months I lived in a nether world of driving up and down to the hospital and sitting next to her incubator, holding her or simply being with her while observing the goings-on in the NICU, seeing babies leave and new babies arrive. All the time I was away from Kate, I felt unreal, in between. I felt real and present only when I was with her. Everything else was preparing, recovering, gearing up for, resting.

Every time you enter the NICU, you have to wash your hands in order to cross the threshold into the sacred place, the place beyond the glass windows, beyond ordinary daily life. Friends came to see Kate when she was a little bigger, and I was allowed to carry her to the window for a few minutes to show her to them. Once, when a dear friend came to see Kate, a nurse who had become quite possessive of her took her away from me and held her up to my friend. I insisted on taking her back into my own arms. As soon as I did so, the nurse insisted that Kate be taken back into the NICU, as she had been out of it long enough. In those first weeks, I had to submit to the authority of the NICU nurses, and had no option but to give Kate back to them when they told me to. I wasn't allowed to hold her for too long in the beginning. When she was sick with a gastric infection in the first weeks, I wasn't allowed to pick her up at all. I could touch her, but only with my hands through the little doors in the side of the incubator. My back and upper arms tired and stiffened from the odd positioning.

Those early months were about existing in the present, not thinking but observing, listening, sitting still, learning a slow, meditative patience while she grew gradually bigger and stronger. Almost imperceptibly she gained a few grams each day and took in a little more milk, while I sat at her side, her attendant mother, guardian angel, witness, nurse. It became a meditation – being there for her.

I remember drinking coffee in disposable cups from the hospital coffee shop. I remember the smell of popcorn, which the nurses often bought to eat at quieter moments. I remember how long the nurses' shifts were – twelve hours. One older nurse told me, 'The best way to be a mother is to learn to trust yourself. Listen to that inner voice. Trust it.' She told me this late one night when we were the only adults in the NICU. All the sick and premature babies were in their cots and incubators, and it was dark and quiet except for a beep now and then and the humming sound from the electronic equipment.

Twice a day I visited Kate, every morning from about eight till about three in the afternoon and then again at night. André bought coal and wood and made a fire in the small Victorian fireplace in our Woodstock home each cold, wet night that winter. Before my night visit I would sit close to the fire in my great-grandmother's chair, deriving comfort from it. I would relax slightly as I stared silently into the flames between mouthfuls of supper, bracing myself for the drive back to the hospital. Our dogs lay next to the fire all night. The wooden floorboards near the fireplace were pocked with black scorch marks from decades of popping coal. I would leave André and the dogs and head out into the rain. Cape Town winter rain is more than just weather – it can feel endless, a permanent submersion, frightening for a non-native. No matter how cold or wet it was outside, as soon as I entered the NICU, I would overheat.

Almost daily, new faces, new mothers arrived. I became a fixture, almost invisible, in my daily vigil. In three days the other women gave birth, got the hang of things, and went out into the world with their babies kitted out in new clothes and receiving blankets, with matching baby bags and new car seats. I stayed on and on. After several weeks of sitting there day after day, I knew most of the routines; I could have acted as an NICU assistant. I remember the nurses gossiping crossly about a twenty-something mother who visited her baby only every two or three days. I also saw that there were far more challenging misfortunes than being premature. There were babies who had to be ventilated; there were babies who were much sicker than Kate. A baby with spina bifida came to the NICU in preparation for a long and highly specialised operation. She was much older than the other babies in the ward.

One of my most traumatic experiences was attempting to breast-feed Kate in the hospital under strict supervision. She had to learn to feed before she could be released from her hospital sentence. I would try and fail. Well-meaning nurses weighed her before and after a feed, and there would be regretful shakes of the head – no, she didn't take anything in. Other nurses, many of whom hadn't ever had a baby of their own, offered me nipple caps, suggested different positions for her head, demonstrated how latching on is supposed to work, but between us all we couldn't get it right. Eventually, thanks to a kind word from an older nurse who had two children of her own, I realised that Kate needed to bottle-feed or we would be in hospital much, much longer. I pumped my breasts, milking myself several times a day, and stored the milk either at the NICU or at home in the freezer. Determinedly, I taught my baby to drink from a bottle.

Kate's first bath was in a two-litre ice-cream container. Before then I washed her body inch by inch with cotton wool and warm water. How light she was and how small, so small she fitted into my hand. I've forgotten, or mostly forgotten, those tiny nappies and knitted caps and what being on red alert was like.

When we brought Kate home, she weighed just two kilograms, still smaller and lighter than most babies are when they are born. I had been deeply apprehensive that I would need to monitor her breathing constantly, that I would need a gadget to tell me that my baby was still alive. But by the time she came home, I trusted the connection between us enough; I knew that she knew how to breathe. She slept in our bed, snuggled between us, and, tiny as she was, I knew that I wouldn't roll over onto her. I had the strangest sensation of both sleeping and being aware of her at the same time, cradled next to my body.

Kate is now five and a half. She delights me every day with her passionate will, that same fighting spirit that was evident from her first moments in the incubator.

Zimanga

Sivuyile Mazantsi

The night before my son was born, I was with my girlfriend, Nomathemba. I was massaging her swollen tummy, a ritual I performed every night. She loved it. I would tell her stories while she lay there, allowing me to feel the fullness of her body. This night, on a Monday in November, I told her a story about a pregnant woman who was making love to her husband. While they were busy, the woman's waters broke and the baby popped out. Not knowing what to do, the husband ran outside naked into the street shouting for help. This is the part Nomathemba really enjoyed.

After I had finished massaging her, I asked her if we could make love to make sure that our child would be born with no missing parts. You know, my folks love this belief – and it is widespread – that every time you make love to your lady during pregnancy, you are certain to add a new part to the unborn baby: an arm, a leg, maybe an ear. The idea entertained her. But she said we could not, as she was afraid the baby would pop out.

Just before I left, she told me she had a craving for snoek. (During her pregnancy, snoek was the only thing Nomathemba craved more than my stories. It was even meatier, she said.) Because the fish shop nearby was closed, I promised to bring her some the next time I saw her.

The following day, on my way home from work, my cellphone rang. It was Nomathemba. 'Please come over,' she said. 'I need you. *And don't forget the snoek.*' She sounded desperate. When I got to her flat, not far from my house, I found her lying on the floor. She was trying hard to breathe through cramps. I gave her the fish, then knelt down and performed my daily ritual – the massage. She asked me if I thought that eating the snoek would bring her some relief. 'Well, there's nothing I can say to that, my

186

love,' I laughed. 'I'm not a doctor.'

Before I left her, at around seven thirty, the cramps had eased. I told her I would be back at nine, but to call me should things get worse. I would ask Noncedo, my housemate, to drive us to the hospital. On my way home I looked at the time on my cellphone. Twenty to eight. I had an appointment with Thembeka. An adorable girl. She was going to treat me to a couple of beers. But something told me that could wait for tomorrow.

I switched on my ghetto blaster and played B.B. King's 'Three o'Clock Blues'. Just before it came to an end, the call came: '*Mmnntwam yy-ii-za ngoku. U-ukude u-nine. Yiza NoNoncedo.*'[1]

Noncedo drove me back to the flat. My girlfriend's sister, Nomalizo, came too. When we got there, Nomathemba was lying where I had left her, moaning. The snoek was still next to her, untouched. Her sister put all the things she thought she would need in hospital into a small bag. Then we sped off in Noncedo's silver-grey Ford Cortina three-litre.

Nomathemba sat in the front passenger seat, groaning. I tried to comfort her, but stopped because I could see my words were just making things worse. She fell silent, and we all quietened. Then she turned to Noncedo. 'Noncedo, you must *never* have a child,' she said, through clenched teeth. Noncedo shook her head. 'Don't worry,' she answered. 'Not yet, anyway. I'm still a student.'

When we arrived at the hospital, Nomathemba found it difficult to walk. 'Be strong. Soon you'll be fine,' Noncedo reassured her. At reception I filled in all the necessary forms, and we were told to take the lift to the second floor. Noncedo could not be with us for long as she had to rush back to finish some schoolwork that was due the following day. So I was left with my girlfriend's sister.

In the maternity section on the second floor, there were many women waiting to deliver. All were screaming in pain.

---

1 'Come now, my love. Nine is too far away. Come with Noncedo.'

Their stomachs came in different shapes and sizes. One of the nurses ushered us to an empty room. She gave Nomathemba maternity pyjamas to wear, and instructed me to help her change. Nomalizo waited outside on a bench.

When we had managed to put on the pyjamas, I accompanied Nomathemba to an examination room. The cramps were getting stronger. The nurse who had given her the pyjamas examined her. She looked at a small TV with graphs moving up and down, and inserted a finger into her private parts. I was shocked, but I lacked the courage to ask why she was doing this. The nurse told me the baby was ready to come out. All this time Nomathemba was screaming in agony, calling my name and begging me not to leave her alone. I promised her I would be there for her.

While gently stroking her to give some comfort, I overheard a nurse telling one of the pregnant women in the room to go home because her time wasn't near. It was hard for me to understand how she could send this woman home, as she was obviously in great pain. Apparently it was the second time they were going to send her away.

Nomathemba had been given a bed and was tossing and turning on it. The nurse who was attending her briefed other nurses about her condition. These nurses walked us to the labour ward, which was not far from the examination room. As we walked down the corridor, I noticed drops of water on the floor. They were coming from Nomathemba. I saw them because I was walking behind her and the nurses. They escorted her the way police escort a prisoner. There was no way she could escape, even if she wanted to. No way.

The nurses did not speak. The only sounds I could hear were screams and moans from the wards we passed. In one ward I saw a fat black woman squatting on the bed.

'*Andimazi lo uyakuzala nini. Kwayizolo ebenje,*'[2] said one of the nurses, referring to the fat woman. My heart started beating like a hammer. Then one of the nurses pointed to Ward Six. That's where the job will be done, I thought to myself.

---

2 'I don't know when this one will deliver. She's been like this since yesterday.'

We entered the ward. The room was big, but there was just one bed. Nomathemba was instructed to lie on her back. Her hands were tied to the frame of the bed. She was told to open her thighs wide apart and then they tied her legs to the lower frame of the bed. One of the nurses was male. I felt so uncomfortable that this guy was seeing my girlfriend naked.

The nurses asked if I would like to remain in the ward when they delivered the baby. I wanted to, but I didn't have the courage to watch the action. They told me where to wait. Instead I went to the reception where Nomalizo was seated and asked her to help me buy baby items at the nearest general dealer. I knew that, being a mother herself, she would know what was needed.

Hardly fifteen minutes had passed before we were back at the hospital. I went straight to the second floor and waited where I was told to, in a small room just outside the delivery ward. I was the only occupant. I looked at my cellphone. It was eleven o'clock. Suddenly, I heard a baby's cry. It came from Ward Six. Then everything went quiet. The only sound I could hear was the monotonous moaning of the fat woman down the corridor. I wanted to phone my friend and let him know that Nomathemba was in the labour ward, but I didn't have airtime. And I didn't know how to send a 'Please call me' message. I hated all this.

After a while I heard footsteps coming towards the waiting room. One of the nurses, a white woman with glasses, appeared at the door and asked me if I was with Nomathemba. 'Yes,' I said. She told me that the delivery was successful, and asked if I could guess the sex of the baby. I told her I didn't mind the sex as long as the baby was healthy. She told me it was a boy and that he was one hundred per cent fit. Then she led me to the ward. The white sheets on my girlfriend's bed were red with blood.

When I saw Nomathemba, she smiled and told me we had a son. The baby was just beside her, wrapped in a bluish blanket and lying in something like a plastic basin. A soul so small. I looked at him and saw myself. 'I'm a father,' I said. Then I bent down and whispered his name to him: 'Zimanga, my son.'

Thirty Fingers, Thirty Toes

Rahla Xenopoulos

I turn the carved wooden latches and lift all the windows, then swing open each slatted shutter sealed by decades of accumulated dust. I stomp happily down the passage, opening the back door and allowing it to creak with the relief of exposure to the sun. I unlock the 'maid's room' and I'm appalled by its size (not much bigger than a writing desk). Standing up on the old toilet with its antiquated chain-flushing mechanism, I open the window grown over with ticky creeper. I open even the garage, with its lingering smell of gasoline and the tools that bear witness to the old man's carpentry hobby.

This house, with the serenity of its funny silence interrupted only by the gentle song of swallows and red-crested barbets, the tap, tap, tapping of crickets and the occasional shouting-out of garbage collectors doing their rounds on a Tuesday morning, none of it, none of it will ever be the same. This house that has stood so calm and so firm with its motionless musty smell of my grandmother's lounge, it shall be rocked to its very foundations. Lockers added in the laundry room for the piles of muddied school clothes, overgrown trees pruned for agile boys to climb, a basketball net hung, garden gate installed, vegetable garden and creeping roses planted. Bigger, wider, deeper, higher, louder, lusher, happier – we are more, we are many, we are abundant!

Sitting on the cracked marble steps of the sun-drenched stoep, I take the time to warn the resident ghosts uncomfortable with change: 'Beware, I come with children! Long may you have lingered in the frangipani trees and the dusty chandelier, but this is our house now. We are in the business of life!'

c

Prior to children, I marked out my life into before being diagnosed with bipolar disorder and after. Prior to that, I outlined my life into before I met Jason and after I met him. Prior to all of that, well, there was a hurly-burly of madness, horror and fun. The euphoria of unmedicated mania, the despair of unmedicated depression, dyslexia, hyperactivity, anorexia, dancing, boyfriends, bulimia, teaching and the odd failed suicide attempt (all this in no particular order). But one thing, one constant throughout my life, was my desire to reproduce.

As the youngest of five children, I always felt horribly deprived of a baby sibling. So much so that I walked all the way down my road knocking on neighbours' doors informing them that my mother was pregnant with Fenster number six and we could not afford to clothe it. Could people please get cracking with knitting? My poor mother was quite stupefied when people arrived unannounced at her front door with booties.

I went through all of my strange incarnations and got myself into all manner of trouble – except, that is, for the pregnancy kind. I met Jason, we fell instantly in love, we moved in together and we got married. But I failed to get pregnant. After I had been diagnosed, medicated and stabilised, my psychiatrist explained the many obstacles and dangers involved in pregnancy. Chemical disorders are hereditary. Having suffered so horribly myself, could I, with a clear conscience, bring a child into the world knowing that it was vulnerable to a chemical disorder? We decided that with our luck the child would, in all probability, be entirely healthy, and, failing this, we decided that the world wouldn't be quite the same without the likes of Sylvia Plath. The fact that I couldn't conceive or carry a child on psychotropic medication didn't deter us. Nor did the dangers of going off medication now that I had finally been stabilised. And then, of course, there was the question of whether I, as a person with a chemical disorder, was really capable of being a competent mother. Would I be able to give a child consistency? We threw caution to the wind and discounted all of these rational fears. Stability was wonderful, but I wanted a baby. Common sense was sensible, but I wanted a baby. What's so great about stability?

Nature's not stable, the weather's not stable. Life's not easy with mental imbalances, but it never fails to challenge. I held out for that baby.

We managed to convince my reluctant psychiatrist, who then cautiously weaned me off my medication. I assured him that I would only do this 'baby thing' once, and then I would resume the life of a cooperative, pill-popping patient. Then the anatomical complications began. I did not get at all pregnant. I did, however, get depressed. I did everything I knew to keep my mood stable. I went to bed every night by ten. I gymmed myself into a daily fervour. I never drank caffeine or alcohol. But when there is a dark cloud hovering over your head, well, it will hover until it descends on your entire being. I got so depressed that I had to be put right back onto all my medication. For a while, I pretended to give up on my dream.

A year later I went off the pills again, only this time with the help of fertility experts. I feel safe with an expert. I'm aware that experts are frequently people with little more than fancy letterheads, but that's of no concern. I myself don't have any expertise – I don't even have much of an education – so I'm confident with the letterheads and the desks with cups of pens. Weeks fell into months, summer into a dark winter, and nothing happened. After many tests and much money spent, two expert experts looked sympathetically into our eyes and explained that Jason and I would never have biological children. Devastated, I panicked. A black cloud came down. I got depressed. And so it was, back onto the safety of medication again.

A year later we tried once more. Only this time we had new experts and new money. We had surgery, harmony, aromatherapy, reflexology, endless yoga, and long walks on the beach. I lived, ate and breathed through the singular obsession of pregnancy. But still, no baby. So, once again, I got sad, really sad. The rose-tinted lenses started to crack and fog over, an awful, dirty shade of helpless grey. I was desolate. So much so, that I made a rather dramatic suicide attempt.

While I was recovering in hospital, a neighbour came and sensibly implored, 'You have a husband who adores you. You can't keep putting him through this. You've tried so hard. Maybe it's too much to ask. Maybe it's time you let it go. Not everyone has to have a child.'

In spite of my sedated, bandaged state, I sat bolt upright and slurred out, 'But I have to have a child. I will not be denied the right to have children. I have sacrificed so much for this stupid sickness, and if I am to be alive it is to be as a mother. I will be a wonderful mother!'

'Yes,' she said. 'I believe you will.'

And so we braved the drama of fertility treatment and the risk of no medication again. Only this time we tried something new. Someone recommended a Chinese doctor. In Los Angeles I'd gone to a Chinese doctor for backache and it seemed to work. Besides which, at this stage I was so desperate I would have taken up tightrope walking. So, one miserable Wednesday, my ever-devoted mother bundled me into Jason's old Jeep and we rattled down the highway as the rain pelted down relentlessly. I arrived – forty minutes late – for an appointment with Professor Zhang. I looked terrible, mottled and chalky, like cellulite, as a result of tension migraines. The only thing capable of numbing the pain was morphine. The professor looked calm and kind, as though he carried with him the wisdom of the Oriental ages. He called his wife, Dr Lee. They felt my pulse, looked at my tongue, and talked to one another in Chinese. They scribbled some symbols onto a notepad, turned me into a pincushion with their mysterious needles, gave me an appalling tea to drink and *sim sala bim BAM BOOM*.

My mother, who had practically carried the chalky apparition into the surgery, was amazed to see her daughter, miraculously restored, breeze back out again. Instantly, I trusted the Chinese doctors. Different people have different forms of medicine that work for them. Maybe it's past-life stuff; maybe it's the interior design of the doctor's reception. I discovered that I was good on a healthy lifestyle, a combination of the right Western drugs and Chinese medicine.

The professor didn't believe my body was ready to hold a child and recommended that I have treatment for six months before trying again. I was nervous about staying off psychiatric medication for so long, but he assured me that they could keep my mood stable, and of course I believed them.

After six months, with the ancient forces of Chinese medicine and the modern marvels of Western science behind us, I went in and tried for another *in vitro* fertilisation. Who knows, maybe it was the needles and the tinctures, or the cylinders and the software. Maybe God got so bored of hearing me nag, of hearing my friends and family praying, day in and day out, that he finally conceded.

The night before we got the results of the blood tests, I couldn't sleep. I said the Shma and the Hail Mary, I prayed to Jah Lord Jah, and I chanted *Om mani padme hum, Om mani padme hum* over and over again.

The next morning I hid. I heard the phone ring. I heard Jason shouting, but I didn't come out. I heard my mother screaming and the dogs barking. Still I hid. Finally, tentatively, I peered around the door at Jason, who said that I was pregnant. I closed the door again, sat on the floor and curled my arms around myself. It was unbelievable. When at last I felt able to emerge, Jason's elated face confirmed the news.

People say you shouldn't announce a pregnancy for the first three months in case anything goes wrong. I knew nothing could go wrong. By midday it seemed everyone in the world knew. By two p.m. every available space in my house, every vase, jam jar, sink and bathtub, was filled; everywhere I looked there were sunflowers in full, glorious, fuck-you cheeky bloom. My neighbour had gone out and bought every single sunflower in Cape Town.

The following day we saw the miracle of a little black dot on a scan. Two weeks later we saw another scan. Only this time it had two little black dots. Halfway through my first trimester, the scan showed not one, not two, but three little black dots. I heard the *doof, doof* and *doof* of three heartbeats confident of their imminent place in the world.

Naturally, doctors expert in the field of multiple births warned us that this was a high-risk pregnancy. Laymen who considered themselves expert in the field of multiple pregnancies warned us that this was a high-risk pregnancy. I scoffed at them all. It was a pregnancy of milk and honey. The colour of Turkish delight. The sound of a young, idealistic Miriam Makeba singing 'Pata Pata'. It was a pregnancy redolent of hope and insanity.

And it was weighty. Every step I took defied the laws of gravity, no small feat considering that Cape Town suffered a heatwave that summer and I lived in a house sixty rough concrete steps up from the road. I stayed put as much as I could, mostly in the splash pool on our deck, gazing out at the wondrous view of the Atlantic Ocean interrupted only by the gigantic form floating before me. I never watched a scary movie or read a disturbing book. It was dreamy. And you know what Madonna says Nietzsche said about dreams: if you want something badly enough, then the whole universe conspires to give it to you!

So it was. Sunday, 27 February 2005. Every piece of literature on parental bonding and mothering instinct speaks of the euphoric moment when they put the soft, helpless newborn on your breast and you feel an instant connection. In my case it didn't happen quite like that. There is a sense of medical urgency about the birth of triplets. For four seemingly endless minutes, frantic doctors and nurses expertly drew life out of my chaotic insides. The first baby out was Gidon. It was Gidon who decided he'd had enough inside and broke my waters. Upon being hauled out of me, he wee'd unceremoniously into the wound. A very teary-eyed Jason put him onto my chest. All around me was utter bloody pandemonium. Doctors, nurses and their assistants were yanking inside me, pushing urgently this way and that. Someone called out, 'We have a girl!' and Layla Tallulah came out. Then I sensed what seemed like a lifetime of trepidation and nerves in the room as they fiddled about trying to dislodge little Samuel Jacob. My emotional husband took Gidon away and said, 'I think you're feeling a little detached.'

Damn right I felt detached! No sooner had the babies been whipped out of my tummy than they were whisked from the theatre to the 'safety' of plastic incubators, to be attached to tubes and ventilators. Come to think of it, the morning of 28

February 2005 swam by in something of a pethidine-induced, blood-deprived haze. It was only at two p.m., when I was wheeled into the hospital nursery, that the world fell into perspective. There lay three teeny-weeny beings, each one under two kilograms. But helpless they were not! From day one they were three feisty individuals.

The nursing staff taught me how to do 'kangaroo care', a more natural form of incubation, where premature babies are tucked under the mother's clothing, against the warmth of her body. At times like this nothing would exist for me except the thump, thump, thumping of three little heartbeats and the feel of minute fingers clutching at my skin, as my babies grasped at their new lives. It's funny to say, but when they were thirty-four weeks old, not due for another six weeks, I admired them. I admired their tenacity and their life force.

And so we bonded.

I am not cured. I still get unreasonably sad, irrationally manic, and occasionally I fly to Joburg where I'm forced to spend weeks in hospital, away from my family, getting my medication tweaked and my mood arranged into something with which I can cohabit. I still go for acupuncture and drink my funny, yucky tinctures. But I live daily with three laughing, living, breathing miracles. They come with the marvel of thirty fingers, thirty toes, six ears, six eyes, three noses, three mouths, and all of them perfectly functioning. I don't know, you've got to believe in God. You've got to believe in something.

Biographical Notes

Troy Blacklaws was born in 1965 in Pinetown, Natal. He began to teach English in East London after two bitter years as a pacifist in the army. Other posts followed in England, Frankfurt and Vienna. He now teaches in Singapore. He has published two novels, *Karoo Boy* and *Blood Orange*.

Roxi Blake was born in Cape Town and studied at the AAA School of Advertising. She has lived in London and New York, and currently works at Ogilvy as a designer.

Elleke Boehmer is Professor of World Literature in English at Oxford University. She has published numerous critical studies and articles on postcolonial writing and the literature of empire, and is the author of three novels: *Screens Against the Sky*, *An Immaculate Figure* and *Bloodlines* (shortlisted for the Sanlam Prize) as well as a novella, *Nile Baby*. A study of Nelson Mandela is forthcoming.

Imraan Coovadia was born in Durban. He graduated with a doctorate in English from Yale and is the author of two novels, *The Wedding* and *Green-Eyed Thieves*, both runners-up for the Sunday Times Fiction Prize. He has also published essays and short stories and is currently working on a new novel. He teaches English Literature at the University of Cape Town.

Willemien de Villiers is an artist and writer. A Fine Arts graduate, she manipulates slip-cast commercial greenware to create unique clay narratives. She has published two novels, *Kitchen Casualties* and *The Virgin in the Treehouse*, as well as several short stories in various collections.

Sandra Dodson has worked as an exhibitions organiser at the Museum of Modern Art in Oxford and the Hayward Gallery in London. Prior to this she studied towards a D.Phil. in English at Oxford University. She has published numerous critical articles, including an award-winning essay on Joseph Conrad's *Lord Jim*. She returned to South Africa in 2003.

Finuala Dowling is a poet, novelist and freelance educational writer. She has published two volumes of poetry, *I Flying* (awarded the Ingrid Jonker Prize) and *Doo-Wop Girls of the Universe* (joint winner of the Sanlam Award). She is also the author of two novels, *What Poets Need* and *Flyleaf*.

Ruth Ehrhardt is training to be a midwife. The story 'Droëland' is a tribute to her mother, Carol Ehrhardt, who was an active union leader and lay midwife on their family farm near Ceres. Ruth is currently working on a biography of her family.

Maire Fisher is a freelance editor and copywriter, and also runs creative writing workshops. Her poetry and short stories have been published in *Twist*, *South Africa Writing*, *Women Flashing* and online by e2k and LitNet. She is currently working on a novel.

Rosamund Haden published her first novel, *The Tin Church*, in 2004. It has since been translated into French, German and Dutch. She has also published children's books, short stories and educational material. She is a freelance writer and editor and is working on her second novel.

Ronel Herrendoerfer is an administrator at a pharmaceutical company. She has one child of her own and has twice acted as a surrogate. She lives in Cape Town.

Joanne Hichens has worked as an artist, lecturer and group facilitator. She co-authored the crime thriller *Out to Score* with Mike Nicol, and is currently working on a crime novel of her own. Her youth novella, *Stained*, is to be published in 2008. She has also written several short stories and articles.

Colleen Higgs is a writer and the founder of Modjaji Books. Her writing has appeared in a range of literary magazines, and she recently contributed a short story to *Dinaane*, an anthology of writing by South African women. She is also the author of the poetry collection *Halfborn Woman*. An advocate of small-scale and self-publishing in South Africa, she worked for many years at the Centre for the Book in Cape Town.

Anneke Kamfer-Sloman is a magazine journalist and writer. She lives in Cape Town with her husband and twin daughters.

Sindiwe Magona is a writer, storyteller and motivational speaker. She is the author of *To My Children's Children* and *Mother to Mother*, optioned by Universal Studios for a film on the life of Fulbright Scholar Amy Biehl.

Sivuyile Mazantsi is from Peddie in the Eastern Cape. He has a BA in Communications from Fort Hare University and has worked at various advertising agencies as a copywriter. He currently runs his own communication consultancy firm in Cape Town.

Epiphanie Mukasano was born in Gisenyi, Rwanda. She taught for two years before studying at the National University of Rwanda, where she graduated with a master's degree in English Literature. In 1994 she fled the country with her husband and children, and has lived in South Africa for nine years. She is published in *Living on the Fence*, an anthology of poetry by refugee women.

Nolubabalo Gloria Ncanywa was born in the Eastern Cape. She joined the HIV support group mothers2mothers in 2002, and was soon afterwards appointed as a Mentor Mother. She subsequently became a Site Coordinator, before being promoted to the head office in Cape Town. She is currently the support administrator to the Regional Manager of mothers2mothers in the Western Cape.

Susan Newham was born in Johannesburg. After years of living and travelling in Thailand, southern Africa, Israel and London, she is now settled in Cape Town. She is an editor of a health magazine and has had numerous articles published in magazines including *Femina*, *Fit Pregnancy* and *Real Simple*. She writes a weekly online column on her experiences as a new mother for *women24*.

Sarah Nuttall is Associate Professor of Literary and Cultural Studies at the Wits Institute for Social and Economic Research (WISER) in Johannesburg. She is the author of *Entanglement: Literary and Cultural Reflections on Post-Apartheid* and editor of *Johannesburg: The Elusive Metropolis*. In 2007 she co-edited the collection *At Risk: Writing on and over the Edge of South Africa*.

Mark Patrick is a paediatrician based at Grey's Hospital, Pietermaritzburg, responsible for child health and outreach in the inland region of KwaZulu-Natal. His work involves developing systems that improve the quality of care received by children in the South African health system.

Albie Sachs is Justice of the South African Constitutional Court. He was a leader in the struggle for human rights in South Africa and a freedom fighter in the African National Congress. He is the author of *The Jail Diary of Albie Sachs*, *The Soft Vengeance of a Freedom Fighter* and *The Free Diary of Albie Sachs*, co-written with Vanessa September. He is also the author of numerous books on issues of gender, the law and human rights.

Reviva Schermbrucker grew up in Johannesburg. Originally trained as an art teacher, she is the author of several children's books, including *Lucky Fish*, *Charlie's House* and *An African*

Christmas Cloth. In addition to writing and illustrating she runs creative writing courses on children's fiction and works as a materials developer for NGOs.

Vanessa September is an urban architect and a member of several boards and committees in the fields of arts and culture and social housing. She is currently working on urban regeneration and public sector projects.

Kholeka Sigenu is a Language Subject Advisor in the Department of Education. She belongs to Women in Writing, a group which empowers women to write and self-publish their work. In 2004 she was winner of a writing competition run by the Centre for the Book and self-published *Ezakowethu*, translated *as Ezakowethu: Folk Stories from Home*.

Marita van der Vyver is a full-time writer of fiction, now living in France. Her many literary awards include the M-Net Prize for *Bestemmings* (*Short Circuits*), the ATKV Prize for *Stiltetyd* (*Time Out*) and the Sanlam Prize for Youth Fiction. Her children's books include *The Hidden Life of Hanna Why*, *Rhenocephants on the Roof* and *Mia's Mom*. Her work has been translated into several languages.

Andrew Weeks was born in Johannesburg. He majored in English and Philosophy at Stellenbosch University, and has a law degree from Wits. He lived in London for almost a decade before returning to South Africa, where he is a lawyer specialising in plain-language contracts.

Tanya Wilson is a clinical psychologist who has run a private psychotherapy practice since 1998, and has contributed to a number of social science research projects over the last ten years. Her clinical work includes psychoanalytic psychotherapy with adults and parents, and play therapy with young children. She has a particular interest in child and infant mental health.

Makhosazana Xaba is a former writing fellow at WISER and the author of a volume of poetry, *these hands*. In 2005 she won the Deon Hofmeyr Award for her short story 'Running'. Originally trained as a general nurse, midwife and psychiatric nurse, she worked for many years as a women's health specialist for both local and international NGOs.

Rahla Xenopoulos has published short stories in magazines and also contributed to the recent anthologies *Women Flashing* and *Twist*. She is currently writing a book of stories inspired by South African paintings.

Phillippa Yaa de Villiers studied mime and theatre in Paris. Since returning to South Africa she has written scripts for television and theatre and worked as a performance poet. In 2005 her play *Where the Children Live* received an audience award and she recently wrote and performed *Original Skin*, which was showcased at the Market Theatre Laboratory. In 2006, she published her first volume of poetry, *Taller than Buildings*.

Acknowledgements

We owe thanks, firstly, to all those who have contributed their personal stories to this collection, and to others who have offered valuable insights, ideas and anecdotes. In addition, special thanks are due to Russell Martin, Maggie Davey and Bridget Impey of Jacana Media, for their enthusiastic response to our proposal and their support throughout; to Lisa Compton, for her skilful copyediting; to Stephen Watson, for his helpful advice; to Anne Schuster and Simone Honikman, for putting us in touch with the refugee writing group and mothers2mothers respectively; to Linda Codron of m2m, for sharing her knowledge; to the National Arts Council and Ben and Shirley Rabinowitz for their generous financial assistance; to Nombulelo Nombewu and Thozama Nqweniso, for giving us time; and finally to our families and friends, for their support, encouragement and tolerance beyond the call of duty.

Other titles by Jacana

A Basket of Leaves:
99 Books that Capture the Spirit of Africa
by Geoff Wisner

African Psycho
by Alain Mabanckou

Khabzela:
The Life and Times of a South African
by Liz McGregor

Coconut
by Kopano Matlwa

The Uncertainty of Hope
by Valerie Tagwira

Moxyland
by Lauren Beukes

Things Without a Name
by Joanne Fedler